13 95

Muir

**The initiation of
the heartbeat**

The initiation of the heartbeat

DENIS NOBLE

Fellow of Balliol College, Oxford
University Lecturer in Physiology

CLARENDON PRESS · OXFORD

1975

Oxford University Press, Ely House, London W. 1

GLASGOW NEW YORK TORONTO MELBOURNE WELLINGTON
CAPE TOWN IBADAN NAIROBI DAR ES SALAAM LUSAKA ADDIS ABABA
DELHI BOMBAY CALCUTTA MADRAS KARACHI LAHORE DACCA
KUALA LUMPUR SINGAPORE HONG KONG TOKYO

CASEBOUND ISBN 0 19 857154 2
© OXFORD UNIVERSITY PRESS 1975

Typeset by E.W.C. Wilkins Ltd., London and Northampton

Printed in Great Britain
by J.W. Arrowsmith Ltd., Bristol

Preface

This book is concerned with the most important oscillator known to man — the heart — and in particular with the electrical mechanisms responsible for initiating the heartbeat. The heart of a healthy person beats about once every second for a period of about 70 years. During a lifetime the heart may therefore beat over 2000 million times. This remarkable performance is offset only by the fact that heart disease is one of the commonest causes of death in modern societies. The investigation of the mechanism of the heartbeat is not only interesting in itself as the study of a fascinating physiological process but may also form the basis of future attempts to develop effective treatments of heart disease.

During the last decade cardiac physiologists have made important advances, and we can now give quantitative accounts of the ionic currents underlying the generation of pacemaker activity and the onset of contraction. However, many of these advances have been made using techniques and methods of analysis that may appear difficult to medical students and clinicians unfamiliar with electronics and mathematics. Yet it is important, if future clinical investigations are to take account of recent physiological work, that the more significant advances should be understood more widely than they are at the present time.

This book was written with this object in mind. It is based on lectures given to second-year medical students and physiology undergraduates at Oxford. All the material has therefore been used in undergraduate teaching, often in the form of circulated lecture notes. Some of the material has already appeared in shorter form in reviews or as chapters of other books. In my own teaching I have felt the need to draw the material together into one book that I hope will be more useful and more readily available to students.

Throughout the book I have tried to be explanatory. I have chosen to describe and, where possible, explain some of the important and difficult features of cardiac excitation within the compass of a relatively short book. This has entailed a high degree of selection. I have not been able to refer to all the important physiological work on the subject done in recent years and, where several groups have been responsible for particular advances, I have chosen to base my account primarily on the work of one of them. The medical student and the clinical investigator are not necessarily interested in a careful assessment of credit and I hope this book will not be used for such a purpose. I am aware of the fact that some of my colleagues in the field may look aghast at some of the short cuts I have taken and others may feel that I have been rather free and, perhaps, arbitrary in my selection of material. My only defence is that to do otherwise would require a much larger book than the one I have chosen to write.

A book of this nature necessarily owes much to students and colleagues who have patiently tolerated my initial attempts to explain recent advances in the subject in undergraduate lectures over the last 10 years. I myself emerge from the process a somewhat wiser man and I hope that some at least of my listeners did too. I am convinced that the most demanding testing ground for scientific explanations lies in the undergraduate theatre, and I count it a great privilege to teach at a University at which all medical students study an honours degree course in Physiological Sciences before proceeding to clinical work. It is to this exacting and highly critical audience that I owe most of the stimulus for writing this book.

Holywell Manor, Oxford   D.N.
March 1975

Acknowledgments

Some of the work described in this book was done in my own laboratory. I should like to acknowledge the support of the Medical Research Council and of the Heart Foundation. It is also a pleasure to acknowledge the help of those who have worked with me. Mr. A.J. Spindler's exceptional skills in micro-engineering have been vitally important. It is difficult to know how to acknowledge this kind of indebtedness but it will be well understood in other biophysical laboratories where the technical engineer is so central to the progress of research. Dr. R.W. Tsien's contribution to the analysis of cardiac potassium currents will be readily apparent to readers of the book. My wife, Susan, and her co-worker Dr. Hilary Brown have been responsible for reminding me that the analysis of cardiac pacemakers does not end with that of the Purkinje fibre. The appropriate chapters of the book will show how important it has become to understand the differences between pacemaker mechanisms in different parts of the heart. I am also indebted to Dr. H. Reuter, Dr. O. Rougier, and Dr. G. Vassort for many valuable discussions on the importance of calcium currents.

I am grateful to the following authors and publishers for permission to reproduce some of the illustrations: The Physiological Society (Figs 2.5, 2.6, 3.4, 4.3, 5.1, 5.2, 5.5, 5.7, 6.6, 6.7, 6.8, 6.9, 6.11, 7.2, 7.3, 7.5, 7.6, 7.7, 8.8, 9.6, 10.1, 10.2); Springer-Verlag (Figs 1.1, 4.1, 4.2, 5.3, 5.4, 5.6, 7.4, 8.4, 9.2); The Royal Society (Fig. 2.4); American Physiological Society (Fig. 6.10); Excerpta Medica (Figs 5.8, 5.9); Society of General Physiologists (Figs 1.3, 2.8, 8.1, 8.3, 8.4); Hans Huber (Figs 1.3, 7.1, 9.4, 9.7, 9.8); Pergamon Press (Fig. 8.2); *Nature* (MacMillans) (Fig. 7.9); Academic Press (Figs 6.1, 6.2, 6.3, 6.4, 6.5); Churchill (Fig. 11.1); American Association for the Advancement of Science (Fig. 8.6); L. Barr (Fig. 2.8); E. Carmeliet (Fig. 5.6); J. Dudel (Figs 4.1, 4.2); H.G. Haas (Fig. 9.2); O.F. Hutter (Figs 1.3, 8.1, 8.2, 8.3, 8.4); A.L. Hodgkin (Figs 2.4, 2.5); C. Ojeda (Fig. 3.3); H. Reuter (Figs 3.4, 4.3, 5.1, 5.2, 5.5, 5.7); W. Trautwein (Figs 1.3, 7.4, 8.1, 8.3, 8.4); M. Vassalle (Fig. 6.10); S. Weidmann (Figs 1.3, 6.2, 7.1, 9.4, 9.7, 9.8, 10.2).

How to use this book

This book has been written to allow the subject to be studied in two different ways, depending on the background knowledge of mathematics possessed by the reader. Although the primary purpose is to describe the significant advances as simply as possible, the problems arising from voltage-clamp work on the heart are not neglected. The mathematics required to discuss these problems has been carefully chosen to provide an introduction to the subject for those who wish to study the quantitative and analytical aspects in further depth. However, in order to allow the non-mathematical reader to use the book, these sections have been placed, wherever possible, at the ends of the relevant chapters. They are marked with a vertical line in the left hand margin to indicate that they may be omitted if desired.

Contents

Contents

1 Introduction

The rate at which the heart beats is variable. It is increased, for example, during exercise and emotional excitement. The frequency of beating is therefore under some form of nervous or hormonal control. However, the origin of the beat lies in the heart itself, which will continue beating regularly even when isolated from the rest of the body and, hence, from all the usual forms of control.

The nature of this autorhythmicity has interested physiologists for a long time (see Brooks and Lu 1972). We do not know who first observed the beating of a completely isolated heart. Such an observation probably occurred incidentally while preparing a slaughtered animal for a prehistoric feast. So far as written records are concerned, we know that Galen (A.D. 129–99) observed the motion of a heart taken out of a living animal (Harris 1973). Leonardo da Vinci (1452–1519) also observed that the heart 'moves by itself' (Bottazzi 1964), and he probably realized that it drives blood into the arteries (see Bayliss 1915). Nevertheless, early views on the purpose and nature of the heartbeat were very confused, and it is an extraordinary fact that Greek scientists first obtained most of the important clues and yet failed to realize that the heart beats in order to circulate the blood. This important discovery was made by Harvey (1628). Fascinating accounts of these historical questions may be found in the books by Whitteridge (1971) and Harris (1973). Even after the discovery of the circulation by Harvey, physiologists could only explain why (i.e. for what purpose) the heart beats rhythmically; the mechanism of the initiation of the rhythm was completely unknown. For many people, the inherent activity of the heart was a major example of the workings of the vital forces thought to be characteristic of living organisms. In fact, the heart was thought by some to be the source of the 'vital spirits', a view which seems to have persisted because of the erroneous belief that the heart was the source of heat in the organism. Although Harvey himself questioned this view and clearly stated that the heart appears to be the source of heat only because the blood it receives is already warm, the controversy continued into the eighteenth and early nineteenth centuries and was only fully resolved

1

when the sciences of physics and chemistry became sufficiently advanced to allow a correct analysis of the origin and flow of heat in animals (see Goodfield 1960). One of the key figures in this development was the French physiologist Claude Bernard whose lifetime (1813–78) saw a complete revolution in physiology and, in particular, the resolution of the mechanist–vitalist controversy, to a large extent as a result of Bernard's own work.

By the end of the nineteenth century, therefore, many of the misconceptions had been cleared and the origin of the heartbeat was an obvious object of study for those interested in the physical and chemical mechanisms of living processes. The end of the nineteenth century was also a time at which confidence in the future success of mechanistic explanations reached a peak. Not that this confidence had not prevailed at times before. Greek scientists had attempted ingenious (though often to us incomprehensible) mechanistic explanations of the heartbeat in terms of thermally induced expansions of fluid in the heart. Aristotle compared it to the process of boiling. Naturally enough, each investigator tried to use the knowledge of physics and chemistry available to him at the time to attempt mechanistic explanations of biological phenomena. The heartbeat was an obvious target for such studies since it is so very clearly a mechanical event and the science of mechanics developed relatively early.

The electrocardiogram

The heartbeat, however, is also an electrical process. Each time the heart muscle contracts, electric currents flow through it. These currents have turned out to be of the utmost importance. They are not incidental accompaniments of mechanical activity, as the currents induced by a moving magnet are. They are the cause of the beat itself. The origin of the heartbeat is an electrical event. A correct investigation of the mechanism therefore required the development of the science of electricity. As we shall see in later chapters in this book, the theory of electrochemistry plays a very large part in our understanding of the behaviour of excitable tissues. The earliest work on the electrical processes occurring in the heart was, of course, descriptive. The detection of these processes relied primarily on the fact that the body in which the heart lies is a salt solution which can conduct electricity. The electric currents generated during beating may therefore be detected in the body a long distance away from the heart itself. They can in fact be detected at the surface of the body (Waller 1887). However, the currents at this distance are very weak, and it was for the purpose of recording these tiny currents that Einthoven (1913) developed the string galvanometer at the beginning of this century. One of his original records is shown in Fig. 1.1.

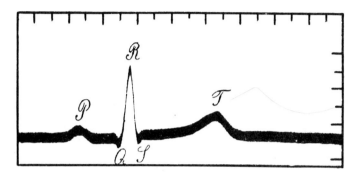

FIG. 1.1. Electrical potentials recorded between the surfaces of the two arms using a string galvonometer. Horizontal scale: time in 50-ms intervals; vertical scale: potential in 0·5 mV intervals. Reproduced from Einthoven (1913).

Each time the heart beats, the potential between two points on the body surface (in this case between the two arms) varies in a characteristic manner. A small slow wave (designated P by Einthoven) is followed after a fast series of changes (Q,R,S) by another slow wave (T). These waves can in fact be associated with events occurring in the heart itself (see p. 10). P corresponds to atrial excitation; Q,R,S to ventricular excitation (depolarization). Moreover, the recording of these waves (called electrocardiograms) on the surface of the body has become important in clinical practice to check whether the heart's activity is normal and to attempt to diagnose cardiac disease. The fact that such records can be obtained quickly with no operative procedure is obviously a great advantage in clinical work.

Unfortunately from the physiologist's point of view, this method of recording the electrical activity of the heart is too indirect and the results that it gives are too complicated to be analysed in terms of ionic current mechanisms. As is frequently the case in scientific research, in order to obtain a result that is simple enough to analyse mechanistically it is necessary to use more elaborate methods. In this case we must record directly from the heart itself, and, preferably, from very small parts of it.

Introduction

Anatomy of heart and conducting system

Before proceeding further with our account, it will be helpful to introduce some elementary anatomy and to define a few important terms used in cardiac electrophysiology. The heart is composed of four chambers. Two of these are large and thick-walled. These are the ventricles, which pump blood into the two main arteries. The right ventricle pumps blood into the pulmonary artery that supplies the lung circulation, and the left ventricle pumps blood into the aorta which supplies the systemic circulation. The other two chambers are small and thin-walled. The right atrium receives blood from the systemic circulation and passes it onto the right ventricle to enter the pulmonary circulation. The left atrium receives blood from the pulmonary circulation and passes it onto the left ventricle to enter the systemic circulation. It is important therefore that the ventricular muscle should be excited after the atrial muscle so that the ventricles are filled as much as possible before ventricular contraction occurs. The correct timing of these events is brought about by the specialized conducting tissues of the heart (see Fig. 1.2). The initiation of electrical activity lies in the sino-atrial (SA) node which is a strip of fine muscle fibres lying near the junction of the superior vena cava with the right auricle. This region (SA node) generates electrical activity spontaneously by a mechanism known as the pacemaker mechanism. It is not the only region of the heart to posess a pacemaker mechanism. However, under normal circumstances, its rate of beating is higher than that of any of the other pacemaker regions so that it sets the pace of the heart as a whole.

The excitation initiated at the SA node spreads through the atrial muscle to produce atrial contraction (the precise nature of the link between electrical and mechanical events in the heart will form the subject of a subsequent chapter – Chapter 5).

In general, the atrial and ventricular muscles are not electrically continuous. Electrical activity in the atrium does not spread across into the ventricle – except at one point: the atrio-ventricular (AV) node. This is a small strip of tissue connecting the two kinds of cardiac muscle. It is composed of very fine fibres that conduct the impulse very slowly to ensure that there is a significant delay between the excitation of the atria and that of the ventricles. Malfunction of this region can lead to excessive delay (shown by an increased time between P and R waves in the electrocardiogram) or to complete failure to conduct. This condition is known as heart-block and is evidenced by P waves occurring

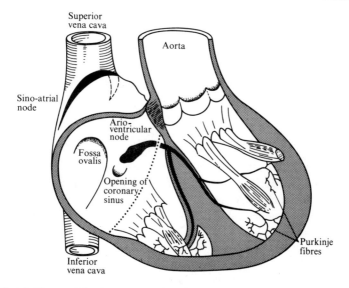

FIG. 1.2. The specialized tissue of the mammalian heart. The pulmonary trunk and part of the right ventricle have been removed. The atrio-ventricular node gives origin to the atrio-ventricular bundle which, in turn ends in the ramifying Purkinje fibre network. (Drawn by Professor E.W. Walls. From Keele and Neil (1965).)

without subsequent Q,R,S, and T waves. Under these conditions the ventricles may fail to contract altogether or they may do so at a fairly slow pace set by pacemaker mechanisms in the conducting fibres beyond the AV node.

These fibres (first carefully described by Purkinje) are large and form the bundle of His that conducts the impulse to the surfaces of the two ventricles. The large size of the Purkinje fibres ensures that the conduction occurs rapidly. (The relation between fibre size and conduction velocity will be discussed in Chapter 2.) The relatively large ventricular muscles are therefore excited almost synchronously, as is essential if their contraction is to suceed in forcing the blood into the arteries at high pressure, rather than simply shifting it between different parts of the ventricle.

Failure to achieve nearly synchronous excitation of the ventricular fibres is therefore a serious condition and occurs when the ventricular activity is desynchronized to cause ventricular fibrillation. The exact cause of ventricular fibrillation is a disputed topic, and I shall discuss possible mechanisms suggested by recent advances in cardiac electro-physiology in Chapter 10.

Ventricular muscle itself does not normally show pacemaker activity and, in conditions of AV block, the beating of the ventricles is probably determined by the relatively slow form of pacemaker activity shown by the Purkinje fibres or fibres of the atrio-ventricular bundle that connects the AV node to the Purkinje fibres.

Cardiac action potentials

The various regions of the heart and the components of the pace-maker and conducting systems are distinguishable anatomically. They are also distinguishable electrically. This may be shown by recording the electrical impulse (or action potential) by fine glass electrodes inserted inside the cardiac cells. The records that may then be obtained are shown in Fig. 1.3.

Record (a) shows spontaneously occurring action potentials recorded from the frog sinus venosus by Hutter and Trautwein (1956). This record is similar to those obtained from the SA node in mammalian hearts. During the action potential, which lasts about half a second, the intra-cellular potential changes from negative to positive. Following the action potential, when a negative potential is restored, the potential spon-taneously changes in a positive direction. This potential change is called the pacemaker potential since it is responsible for initiating another action potential when the depolarization reaches the excitation threshold (Arvanitaki 1938; Bozler 1943). Variations in the rate of the heartbeat are largely brought about by variations in the rate of potential change during the pacemaker potential (see Chapter 8).

There is no hard and fast distinction between sino-atrial node tissue and atrial tissue proper. Atrial tissue lying close to the SA node (or to the sinus venosus in the frog) also shows pacemaker activity, and the records obtained are similar to those in the SA node, although the frequency is lower. From an electrophysiological point of view, there-fore, the SA node is identified as that region of the atrium where the spontaneous firing generated is at its highest frequency. As we move away from the SA node, however, the electrical properties of the tissue change, and it is found that large parts of the atrium are naturally quiesc-ent and fire only when excited either by waves conducted from the SA node or by electrical current stimuli applied artificially. The record then obtained is illustrated in record (b), which was obtained from a dog atrium by Hoffman and Suckling. Notice that there is no spontaneous pacemaker

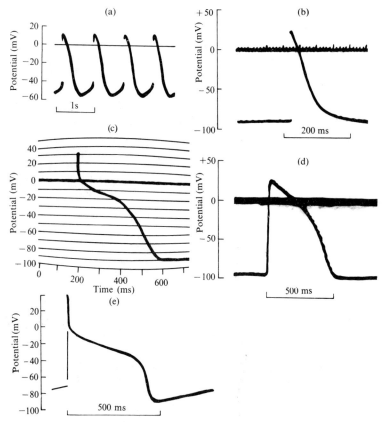

FIG. 1.3. Action potentials and pacemaker activity recorded in different parts of the heart. The natural pacemaker, the SA node or sinus venosus (a), is sponta- neously active and the membrane potential never becomes more negative than -60 mV. Each action potential is followed by a slow spontaneous depolarization known as the pacemaker potential. The atrium (b) has a higher resting potential (which may be up to -80 mV or -90 mV), and a triangular-shaped action poten- tial. It is usually quiescent, although pacemaker activity can be induced by steady depolarizing currents (see Fig. 7.8, p. 100). Purkinje fibres are sometimes quiescent (c) and sometimes show pacemaker activity (e). This pacemaker activity occurs at very negative potentials (-90 to -70 mV) below the range at which sinus pace- maker activity occurs. The action potential shows two phases of fast repolarization separated by a very slow phase known as the plateau. The ventricular fibres (d) have a much higher plateau and show no pacemaker activity. (a) Recorded from frog sinus venosus (Hutter and Trautwein 1956). (b) Recorded from dog atrium by Hoffman and Suckling (from Weidmann 1956). (c) Recorded from dog Purkinje fibre by Draper and Weidmann (1951) (photograph from Folkow and Neil (1971).) (d) Recorded from frog ventricle by Hoffman (from Weidmann 1956). (e) Recorded from sheep Purkinje fibre (Weidmann 1956).

7

activity (the potential is quiescent following the action potential) and that the resting value of the membrane potential is more negative (about −80 mV) than the maximum negative potential achieved during spontaneous activity in pacemaker tissue (about −60 mV). This suggests that the presence or absence of pacemaker activity may depend on the level of the membrane potential following each action potential. This is indeed the case. As will be shown in a later chapter (Chapter 7), quiescent atrial tissue may be made to develop pacemaker activity simply by lowering the resting potential artificially with applied currents.

Records (c) and (e) show electrical activity recorded from the Purkinje fibres of the conducting system. The action potential in these fibres is characteristically different from those in atrial tissue. The initial positive potential rapidly diminishes towards zero potential, and the potential then moves very slowly towards more negative values. This very slow phase of repolarization is known as the plateau phase. It is terminated by a more rapid phase that restores the membrane potential to about −90 mV. In the case of record (c) the potential then rests at −90 mV until the next excitation arrives, i.e. the fibre is quiescent until stimulated. Record (e) shows an example of pacemaker activity in the Purkinje fibre system. Note that, unlike that in the sino-atrial region, the pacemaker potential occurs at very negative potentials. The maximum negative potential at the beginning of the pacemaker potential is −90 mV which is the same as the resting potential in the quiescent fibre (c). In the case of Purkinje fibres, therefore, the presence or absence of pacemaker activity is not simply dependent on the level of the membrane potential following each action potential. These differences suggest that there may be important differences between the pacemaker mechanisms in the atrium and in the conducting system. This is indeed the case, as will be shown in Chapters 7 and 8.

Finally, record (d) shows an action potential recorded from ventricular muscle. In this case, there is also a 'plateau' during which repolarization occurs very slowly but it starts at the peak of the action potential. There is no very rapid initial phase of repolarization. Note also the absence of pacemaker activity. Ventricular muscle in adult tissue is normally quiescent until stimulated by the Purkinje fibres or by applied artificial stimuli.

Notice that in all regions of the heart the action potential lasts for a significant fraction of a second. The shortest action potential (record (b)) lasts nearly 200 ms, while the longer duration action potentials last more than 500 ms. These durations are characteristic of action potentials in cardiac muscle (Burdon-Sanderson and Page 1883), and they contrast very markedly with those recorded in nerve fibres and in skeletal muscle which are typically only one or a few milliseconds in duration.

This difference is related to an important respect in which the electrical events in the heart differ from those in skeletal muscle in function. In skeletal muscle, the action potential is simply a trigger for mechanical activity. Indeed, as shown in Fig. 1.4, the action potential in skeletal

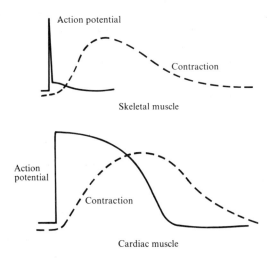

FIG. 1.4. Comparison between relative time scales of electrical (continuous curve) and mechanical (interrupted curve) activity in skeletal and cardiac muscle.

muscle is virtually over before the mechanical response begins. By contrast, the action potential in heart muscle lasts almost as long as the contraction phase. In consequence, the action potential may act not only as a trigger for the initiation of contraction. It may also control its duration and magnitude. This may be demonstrated by artificially shortening or prolonging the action potential by applied current (Morad and Trautwein 1968). Shortening the action potential reduces the magnitude and duration of contraction while prolonging the action potential has the opposite effect.

The long-lasting nature of the action potential in the heart also serves another purpose; the cells do not become excitable again until the action potential is terminated. This period of inexcitability is called the refractory period. In nerve, it lasts about 1 ms, which corresponds to the duration of the nerve action potential, whereas in cardiac muscle it lasts several

9

hundred milliseconds. This long refractory period prevents the muscle being re-excited until the previous contraction is largely over. This is obviously important in a muscle that acts as a pump. There is no function for tetanic (i.e. maintained) contractions in the heart, indeed their occurrence would be disastrous since the ventricle would stay contracted and cease to pump. The long refractory period is also an important factor in preventing fibrillation (see Chapter 10).

Relation of electrocardiogram to action potentials

Although this book is concerned primarily with explaining the mechanisms of intracellular potential changes, it may be helpful to readers interested in clinical applications to know how the changes are related to those of the electrocardiogram. A full treatment of the subject of extracellular fields during cardiac activity is highly complex and beyond the scope of this book. We shall instead limit ourselves to describing the correlations between intracellular action potentials and the extracellular electrocardiogram and to giving a highly simplified explanation for these correlations.

This may best be done by observing the temporal relations between intracellular and extracellular records obtained simultaneously from the same heart. Such an experiment is illustrated in Fig. 1.5. The records were obtained during a demonstration on a tortoise heart performed by Jean Banister and myself to an undergraduate class in 1969 and, as its purpose was entirely didactic, the experiment suits the purpose of this account very well. Four records are shown. The top record is the intracellular record from the atrial muscle. The second record is the extracellular electrocardiogram which we chose to record from the surface of the atrium. This record is similar to that obtained by Gotch (1910) from the surface of a tortoise heart. As will be made clear below, the results differ in some respects from the classical electrocardiogram recorded from the surface of the body (Fig. 1.1) but they are fairly easy to relate to the classical electrocardiogram. The third record shows the intracellular changes recorded in the ventricle and the fourth record shows the first time derivative ($\partial V/\partial t$) of the ventricular record. The purpose of including this record will become evident later.

First, we may note the important differences between an electrocardiogram from the surface of the heart and that obtained from the surface of the body. The waves in the record shown in Fig. 1.5 (b) have been labelled 1,2,3, and 4. Wave 1 corresponds to wave P of the classical record (see Fig. 1.1) but is relatively much larger. The reason for this

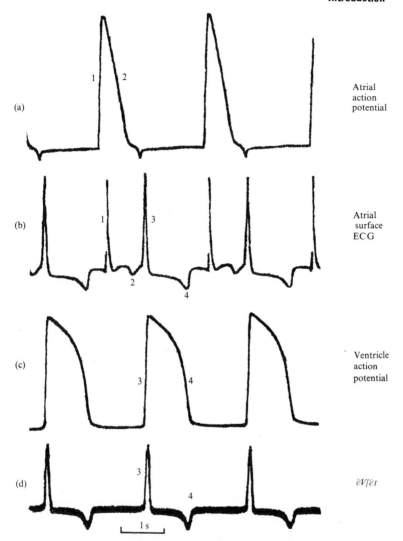

FIG. 1.5. Relations between intracellular action potentials and extracellular electro-cardiogram in tortoise. (a) Atrial action potential recorded with a suction electrode. 1, depolarization: 2, repolarization. The dip following each action potential is an artefact caused by ventricular excitation. (b) Atrial surface electrocardiogram. The waves labelled 1 and 2 correspond in time to atrial events (a). Those labelled 3 and 4 correspond to ventricular events (c). (c) Ventricular action potential recorded with a suction electrode. 3, depolarization; 4, repolarization. (d) Differential ($\partial V/\partial t$) of ventricular record. Note resemblance to ventricular components of electrocardiograms.

11

difference is simply that the record is taken from the surface of the atrium rather from that of the body. As a result the rather weak currents of the thin atrial muscle are recorded at full strength near their source, whereas those of the ventricle are attenuated by the fact that they are recorded at a distance from their source. In the classical electrocardiogram, of course, the atrial and ventricular components are subject to similar attenuation factors since they are at roughly equal distances from the body surface. Moreover, since the atrial muscle mass is much smaller than that of the ventricle, the atrial component of current (P) is smaller. The second major difference is that, in the tortoise cardiac surface record, wave 4 is a negative wave, whereas the T wave of the classical record to which it corresponds, is normally a positive wave. The possible reasons for this difference will be discussed later.

It is a simple matter now to correlate the phases of the intracellular records. Wave 1 ($\equiv$ P in classical record) corresponds to atrial depolarization. Wave 2 (to which there is no correlate in the classical record) corresponds to atrial repolarization. The absence of a wave like this in the classical electrocardiogram is not surprising. It is a very small wave and, as already noted above, is relatively larger in this record than it would be in a classical record. In the classical electrocardiogram it would be insignificantly small and probably lost in the beginning of the QRS complex. Wave 3 ($\equiv$ QRS in classical record) clearly corresponds to ventricular depolarization and wave 4 ($\equiv$ T) to ventricular repolarization. The interval between 1 and 3 ($\equiv$ PR interval) gives the delay between atrial and ventricular excitation and that between 3 and 4 ($\equiv$ RT interval) gives the duration of depolarization in the ventricle, i.e. the duration of the ventricular action potential.

These conclusions may be drawn simply from inspection of the records. The question why the extracellular record takes the particular form it does requires further explanation. The extracellular record measures potentials generated by extracellular current flow during the action potential. A full analysis of extracellular fields is necessarily complex (Geselowitz and Schmitt 1969). However, the major features of the extracellular record may be explained by noting that extracellular current flow depends on potential differences occurring between different parts of the heart. If all cells in the heart fired at exactly the same time and followed the same shape of action potential there would be no spatial variations in potential and no extracellular current flow. However, this is not the case and, as the action potential spreads from one part of the heart to another, voltage gradients are generated. We shall discuss the quantitative aspects of voltage gradients and spread of excitation in more detail in Chapters 2 and 4. For the present account it is sufficient to use one important result. This is that the density of intracellular axial current flow (i_a) along a fibre is proportional to the voltage gradient along it, i.e.

$$\partial V/\partial x = r_a i_a \quad \dagger \qquad (1.1)$$

(see eqn (2.10)), where V is the intracellular voltage and r_a is the resistance to axial current flow per unit length.

If the action potential conducts at a constant speed (obviously an approximation in a complex tissue like the heart) the distance x travelled by the wave in a given time t is determined by the conduction velocity θ, so that

$$\theta \frac{\partial V}{\partial x} = \frac{\partial V}{\partial t} , \qquad (1.2)$$

i.e. the spatial gradients generating i_a are large when the time derivative is large. Hence

$$i_a = \frac{1}{r_a \theta} \frac{\partial V}{\partial t} . \qquad (1.3)$$

This equation is obtained by replacing $\partial V/\partial x$ by $(1/\theta)(\partial V/\partial t)$ in eqn (1.1) and then rearranging to obtain an expression for i_a. Thus we show that i_a is proportional to $\partial V/\partial t$.

Finally we may note that it is the density of extracellular current that determines the magnitude of the electrocardiogram and this must be proportional to the intracellular current flow i_a, since, together with the cell membranes, the extracellular and intracellular fluids form a closed circuit round which the current flows. The extracellular current, and the extracellular potentials recorded in the electrocardiogram, will also therefore be proportional to the first time derivative of the intracellular potential changes.

These expectations are tested in the fourth record shown in Fig. 1.5, which shows the ventricular action potential after it has been processed by an electronic differentiator to give a record proportional to $\partial V/\partial t$. The result is strikingly similar to the ventricular component of the

---

$\dagger$ Equation (1.1) is a form of Ohm's law. It is obtained by relating the voltage change δV across a distance δx, to the product of the current i_a, and the resistance $r_a \delta x$.

electrocardiogram.[†] Similarly, it may now be clear that the atrial component is related to the first derivative of the atrial action potential. This rather simplified analysis leaves one important feature of the classical electrocardiogram completely unexplained. This is that the T wave is normally, though not always, a positive wave, whereas if the electrocardiogram were simply related to $\partial V/\partial t$, it would be a negative wave, as in Fig. 1.5.

The explanation for this phenomenon may lie in the fact that the action potential does not follow exactly the same time course in different parts of the ventricle. If action potentials are recorded at the tip (apex) of the ventricle they are usually found to be significantly shorter in duration than those recorded at the base (i.e. near the AV node). The reasons for this difference are unknown, but it might be attributable to very small variations in extracellular potassium concentrations to which the action potential duration is very sensitive (see Chapter 9).

Whatever its explanation, this difference means that the part of the ventricle that is excited last repolarizes first. The wave of repolarization therefore travels in the opposite direction to that of excitation. The sign of the conduction velocity is therefore reversed and the sign of i_a in eqn (1.3) is changed. The extracellular potential change becomes a positive wave rather than a negative one.

This point is illustrated in Fig. 1.6, which shows how the difference between the base and apex action potentials may resemble the classical electrocardiogram when the apex action potential is shorter than that at the base. The sign of the T wave is one of the features of the electrocardiogram that is of clinical interest. Inversions of the T wave may indicate disturbances in the pattern of spread of repolarization in the ventricle.

Finally, it is worth noting that no reference has been made in this account to electrocardiogram components corresponding to the spread of activity in the specialized conducting system of the heart. The reason is a very simple one: no such components are detectable. The conducting system forms a very small fraction of the cardiac mass and the currents it generates are negligible by comparison with those generated by the atrium and ventricle. The activity of the conducting system may therefore be deduced only indirectly from the timing of the atrial and

---

[†] It is worth repeating the point that this analysis neglects some important features. Thus the classical ECG contains a *triphasic* wave (QRS) corresponding to ventricular depolarization, whereas the explanation given here can only account for a *monophasic* wave (wave 3).

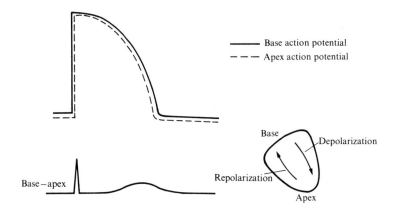

FIG. 1.6. Top diagram shows action potentials at base and apex of ventricle showing the apex to be excited last and repolarizing first. Lower diagram shows difference between top records. Right: direction of depolarization and repolarization waves. (Note: this diagram illustrates only one of several ways in which negative T waves may be produced.)

ventricular components. Thus the interval between the P and R waves may be used to measure the time for atrio-ventricular conduction, most of which corresponds to the delay in conduction in the AV node.

2 Theory of electric current flow in excitable tissues

In subsequent chapters I shall describe the ionic currents responsible for the potential changes described in Chapter 1. These ionic currents are analysed using methods introduced by Hodgkin and Huxley in 1952. The purpose of this chapter is to explain these methods and the background physico-chemical theory involved. I shall do this by discussing the various factors that control the ionic current flow and how the ionic currents in turn generate the action potential.

Ion concentration gradients and ion pumps

The species of ions that carry most of the current flow across cardiac cell membranes are sodium (Na^+), calcium (Ca^{2+}), potassium (K^+), and chloride (Cl^-). In each case, the intracellular concentrations are very different from the extracellular concentrations. The sodium and potassium concentration gradients run in opposite directions and are maintained by the Na^+–K^+ exchange pump that accumulates K^+ inside the cell and keeps the intracellular concentration of Na^+ low. The Na^+–K^+ exchange pump is important in all excitable cells since the resting potential is primarily determined by the K^+ concentration gradient and sodium ions are usually responsible for the depolarization phase of the action potential. So far as cardiac muscle is concerned we may note three important properties of the pump that will be relevant to the interpretation of both normal and pathological behaviour.

1. The pumping rate is steeply dependent on the extracellular K^+ concentration below a certain level. At low K^+ concentrations, therefore, the Na^+ concentration gradient will be K^+-dependent. Moreover, since the Ca^{2+} gradient is dependent on the Na^+ gradient (see p. 17 below), the calcium gradient may also be K^+-dependent. Variations in plasma K^+ are common, and sometimes severe, in certain cardiac diseases, particularly those associated with renal malfunction. It is conceivable that some of the cardiac disturbances in these cases are secondarily produced by hypokalaemia (low-

plasma K^+). The level of plasma K^+ has a large effect on the electrical activity of the heart, though it is likely that most of this effect is attributable to changes in K^+ conductance rather than to changes in ionic pumping over physiological ranges of plasma K^+ (2 mM to 5 mM). These effects will be discussed in Chapter 9.

2. The cardiac glycosides, digitalis and ouabain, are specific blockers of the Na^+-K^+ pump. Digitalis (usually as digoxin) is widely used in clinical practice to treat heart-failure. It is still not clear whether or how its restorative action on a failing heart is related to its action on the Na^+ pump, though it is possible, once again, that the secondary dependence of the calcium gradient on sodium pumping may be involved (see Chapter 5).

3. In most excitable cells it has been found that the pump moves more sodium ions than potassium ions. It tends therefore to carry net positive charge from the inside of the cell and so hyperpolarize it, i.e. the activity of the pump may contribute directly to the negative intracellular potential. Isenberg and Trautwein (1974) have shown that cardiac glycosides reduce the outward current in Purkinje fibres (see p. 121).

The existence of the Na^+-K^+ pump has been established for a long time. It is only relatively recently that the existence of Ca^{2+} pumps has been demonstrated. Two mechanisms appear to exist. The first is a direct outward Ca^{2+} pump involving the use of energy from ATP. The second is an outward movement dependent primarily on the Na^+ concentration gradient and appears to derive its energy from this gradient. It is therefore secondarily dependent on the Na^+-K^+ pump. The evidence for these pumps in a variety of tissues has been reviewed recently by Baker (1972). In the case of excitable cells the Na^+-dependent Ca^{2+} pump appears to be the most important and it has been clearly demonstrated in cardiac muscle (Lüttgau and Niedergerke 1958; Niedergerke 1963; Reuter and Seitz 1968; Glitsch, Reuter, and Scholz 1970).

Unlike the Na^+-K^+ pump, the Na^+-Ca^{2+} pump is not blocked by cardiac glycosides. The dependence on external sodium ions is very specific. The very similar ion Li^+, which is accepted by the Na^+ conductance mechanism in excitable cells, will not substitute for sodium ions in the pump mechanism.

In the case of calcium ions, there is a further factor to be taken into account that determines the concentration gradients, and which is also very important in relation to the role of calcium ions in the initiation of contraction. Unlike the monovalent cations Na^+ and K^+, which are largely free, the majority of intracellular Ca^{2+} is in a bound or sequestered form. Part of this binding may be attributable to Ca^{2+} binding sites on intracellular proteins but the great majority is attributable to Ca^{2+} uptake by internal membranous organelles such as mitochondria or the sarcoplasmic reticulum. Since the fraction of Ca^{2+} bound in this way is very large, minor variations in uptake may have a large effect on the intracellular calcium concentration. This may be particularly important in cardiac muscle since the uptake and release mechanisms are probably controlled by drugs like adrenaline that are important in the natural control of cardiac function. They may also be affected by the cardiac glycosides.

Finally, there is some evidence that chloride ions may be actively transported into cardiac cells. The estimated intracellular chloride concentration is somewhat larger than would be expected if chloride ions moved purely passively across the membrane.

Fig. 2.1 summarizes the ion pumps in cardiac cells and gives typical

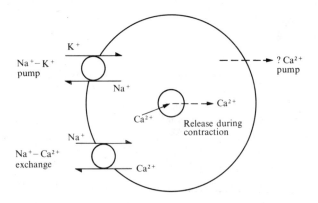

	Intracellular	Extracellular
Na^+	30 mM	140 mM
K^+	140 mM	4 mM
Ca^{2+}	100 nM	2 mM
Cl^-	30 mM	140 mM

Ion concentrations

FIG. 2.1. Ion movements due to pumps (above) and typical ion concentrations (below).

values of the various ion concentrations. These values may now be used to estimate the electrochemical gradients acting on the various ion species.

Electrochemical potential gradients

In the absence of an electric potential across the cell membrane, the movement of ions of a given species would be determined simply by the concentration gradients and membrane permeability. Thus, potassium ions would diffuse out of the cell. In the presence of a negative intracellular potential tending to attract positive ions, this loss will be reduced or reversed depending on whether the electrical force moving ions into the cell is smaller or larger than the concentration gradient moving ions out. The algebraic sum of these two forces, which determines the net flow, is called the electrochemical potential gradient. This gradient is zero when the two forces are equal and opposite. There is then no net flux and the system is in equilibrium. The potential at which this occurs, the equilibrium potential, is given by the Nernst equation:

$$E = \frac{RT}{zF} \ln \frac{[C]_o}{[C]_i}, \tag{2.1}$$

where R is the gas constant, T the absolute temperature, z the valency of the ionic species involved, F is the Faraday, and $[C]_o$ and $[C]_i$ are the extracellular and intracellular ion concentrations. Thus, for potassium ions we obtain (using the values in Fig. 2.1)

$$E_{K^+} = \frac{RT}{F} \ln \frac{4}{140} = 61 \log \frac{4}{140} = -94 \text{ mV}, \tag{2.2}$$

since $RT/F = 26$ mV at $37°$C and $\ln x = 2 \cdot 303 \log x$. Similarly, we obtain $E_{Na^+} = +41$ mV, $E_{Ca^{2+}} = +133$ mV and $E_{Cl^-} = -41$ mV.

It should be emphasized that although these values are typical ones they are not constants *in vivo*. The ionic concentrations are dependent on a variety of factors, some of which have already been mentioned in this chapter. Variations in ionic concentrations produce corresponding variations in the equilibrium potentials.

When the membrane potential is not equal to the equilibrium potential, there will be a net flow of ions determined by the difference between the membrane potential and the equilibrium potential. Thus, for potassium ions the current i_{K^+} carried will be given by

$$i_{K^+} = g_{K^+}(E - E_{K^+}), \tag{2.3}$$

19

where g_{K^+} is the membrane conductance to potassium ions.[†] As we shall see below, this conductance is dependent on the number of conducting channels in the membrane as well as on the properties of the individual channels. Variations in the numbers of conducting channels occur throughout the action potential, and to describe these variations Hodgkin and Huxley introduced the gating variables described below (see p. 22). Since it is useful to be able to refer to the conducting properties of the ion-transfer process itself, they also introduced the parameter $\bar{g}$ to refer to the conductance that obtains when *all* the channels are conducting (i.e. when the gating mechanism is fully open). We may refer to the current carried under these conditions as $\bar{i}$. Thus, for potassium ions,

$$\bar{i}_{K^+} = \bar{g}_{K^+}(E - E_{K^+}). \tag{2.4}$$

The variation of $\bar{i}_{K^+}$ with membrane potential then describes the property of the ion-transfer process itself independent of any gating mechanism that may operate.

Hodgkin and Huxley's (1952) work on the squid giant nerve axon suggests that the ion-transfer process is a very simple one. The conductances $\bar{g}_{K^+}$ and $\bar{g}_{Na^+}$ were found to be constants, as would be expected if the ionic channels behaved as simple ohmic conductors. The ionic current is then a linear function of the driving force $(E - E_{K^+})$.

However, in cardiac muscle membrane, as indeed in other excitable cells apart from the squid axon, the ion-transfer processes have been found to be more complex.

The ion-transfer process

Frankenhaeuser (1962) showed that in frog myelinated nerve the outward K^+ current in response to a large depolarization (of the order of 100 mV) is considerably greater than would be expected if the potassium channels behaved as linear conductors. The channels therefore conduct more easily as outward current is passed through them. This phenomenon is known as *outward-going rectification* since the channels behave as rectifiers passing outward current better than inward current.

In the case of cardiac muscle some at least of the K^+ channels show behaviour of the opposite kind, i.e. the channels pass outward current in response to positive potential changes less easily than they pass

---

[†] This equation is based on Ohm's law. This may be clear when it is noted that the conductance g is the reciprocal of resistance r. Thus, eqn (2.3) might also be written: $E - E_{K^+} = i_{K^+} r_{K^+}$, where r_{K^+} is the resistance to the flow of potassium ions.

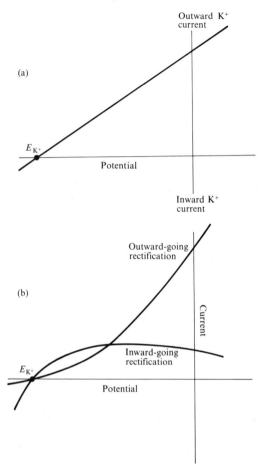

FIG. 2.2. (a) Current–voltage diagram for K^+ channels whose current is a linear function of potential. Note that the current is zero at E_{K^+}. (b) Current–voltage diagrams for channels showing outward-going and inward-going rectification.

inward current in response to negative potential changes. They are therefore said to show *inward-going rectification* (see Fig. 2.2).

The mechanisms of the ion-transfer processes that produce this kind of behaviour are still uncertain (for discussions of possible mechanisms see Adrian (1969), Armstrong (1971), and Jack, Noble, and Tsien (1975, Chapter 8). Whatever the mechanisms, the existence of inward-going rectification in the K^+ channels of cardiac muscle has very important consequences. The total ion movements during the action potential are considerably smaller than they would be in the absence of inward-rectification. The properties of the inward-rectification process are also crucially important in determining the changes produced by variations in extracellular potassium concentrations. In view of the clinical importance of the effects of plasma K^+ changes, I shall discuss them in some detail in a later chapter (Chapter 9).

Ion gating mechanisms

In the resting state, at potentials near -80 mV, very few of the total number of ionic channels are found to be conducting. As the membrane potential is varied in a positive (depolarizing) direction the fraction of open channels increases. The channels are therefore controlled by a voltage-dependent gating mechanism. The response of this mechanism to an instantaneous voltage change is not instantaneous. A certain period of time is required for the mechanism to change to a new steady state. The gating mechanisms therefore introduce both voltage and time-dependence in the ionic current.

Since Hodgkin and Huxley first analysed the kinetics of the gating mechanisms in squid **nerve** membrane, various alternative kinetic schemes have been proposed, some of which have proved as successful as – or even more so than – that of Hodgkin and Huxley. It is of course important, so far as the study of the chemical mechanisms is concerned, to determine which kinetic schemes are correct, but from a physiological point of view this question is not so important. Provided the kinetic scheme chosen adequately describes the voltage-and time-dependence of the ionic current, it may be used to determine how the ionic current changes generate the normal electrical activity observed. The Hodgkin–Huxley scheme is one of the simplest and for explanatory purposes I shall use it in this account.

Fig. 2.3 shows a schematic version of the model. Each channel is controlled by a charged 'gate' that may occupy either of two positions. In one position α the gate is open and allows the channel to conduct. In the other position β the channel is blocked. A first-order reaction is assumed between these two states. If the fraction of gates in the α state is y, the fraction in the β state will be $1-y$. If the opening **rate coef**ficient is α_y and the closing rate coefficient β_y the rate of opening will be given by $\alpha_y(1-y)$ and the rate of closing will be $\beta_y y$. The net rate of change dy/dt in the fraction of open channels will therefore be given by

$$dy/dt = \alpha_y(1-y) - \beta_y y. \tag{2.5}$$

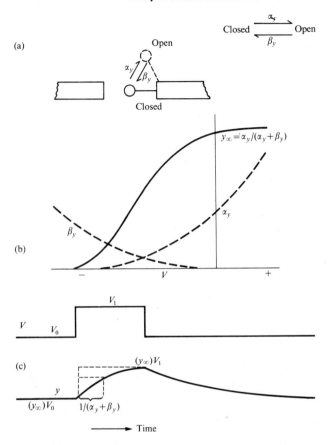

FIG. 2.3. Schematic diagram of Hodgkin–Huxley mechanism for voltage and time dependence of ionic current flowing through a channel. (a) The two states of the gating mechanism. (b) The steady-state activation curve y_∞ and the opening (α_y) and closing (β_y) rate coefficients as functions of potential. (c) Response of y to a step change in potential. The time required for $\frac{2}{3}$ of change to occur is $1/(\alpha_y + \beta_y)$.

Since the gating structure is charged, its tendency to move into the open or closed positions will be voltage-dependent. Since depolarization opens the channels, α_y must increase on depolarization. Similarly, β_y must decrease. In the steady state, $dy/dt = 0$ and the steady-state value y_∞ may be obtained by setting eqn (2.5) to zero and rearranging to give

$$y_\infty = \alpha_y/(\alpha_y + \beta_y). \tag{2.6}$$

23

Theory of electric current flow in excitable tissues

As shown in Fig. 2.3, y_∞ is a sigmoid function of membrane potential. This curve is usually called the activation curve since it determines the degree of activation of the ionic current channels. The voltage at which y_∞ first becomes large enough to detect the ionic current is called the activation threshold.

The current i_y carried by the channels will be given by the maximum current $\bar{i}_y$ (cf. eqn (2.4) above) multiplied by the fraction of channels conducting. Hence

$$i_y = y\bar{i}_y. \tag{2.7}$$

This is the form of equation for ionic current that will be used in later chapters.

When the potential is changed suddenly from one value to another, the value of y will change following an exponential time-course which is the solution to eqn (2.6) when α_y and β_y are constants (see Fig. 2.3). The time-constant for this process is equal to $1/(\alpha_y + \beta_y)$. Some of the current mechanisms in cardiac muscle are found to show exponential changes following step changes in potential (see Chapters 6 and 7). Equations like (2.7) can then be used without modification. However, the current mechanisms in squid nerve, and those for some of the cardiac components, do not behave quite so simply.

Application of theory to squid nerve

The onset of K^+ current in squid nerve was found to follow a sigmoid time-course, not an exponential one. Hodgkin and Huxley showed that this phenomenon could be explained by supposing that more than one gating mechanism operates each channel. If all the gates must be open for the channel to conduct, the probability that the channel will conduct will then be determined by y^γ, where γ is the number of gates involved. This point may readily be tested by supposing that two gates are involved. When $y = 0.5$, i.e. half the gates are open, there will be four equally probable states: both gates open; one open and one closed; the first gate closed and the second one open; both gates closed. Of these, only one state is conducting, i.e. both gates open. The fraction of conducting channels will therefore be 0.25, which is 0.5^2.

The K^+ current in squid nerve was fitted by the equation

$$i_{K^+} = n^4 \bar{g}_{K^+}(E - E_{K^+}), \tag{2.8}$$

where n is the y-variable for the K^+ channels and there are four gates operating each channel. The precise value of γ is not certain. Later work

24

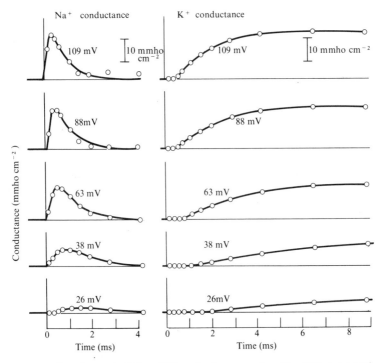

FIG. 2.4. The changes in Na⁺ and K⁺ conductances produced by different magnitudes of depolarization. The depolarization is shown by the number on each curve (Hodgkin 1958). The points are experimental values. The lines are given by Hodgkin–Huxley theory.

on squid nerve suggests that a value larger than 4 may be more accurate, while in myelinated nerve, Frankenhaeuser found $\gamma = 2$. As already noted, some of the cardiac currents are fitted by exponential time-courses, for which $\gamma = 1$. There is clearly a wide degree of variation in the quantitative properties of the gating mechanisms.

The fitting of the theory to the Na⁺ current records introduces a further complication. The increase in Na⁺ current during depolarization is not maintained. Following its relatively fast onset it decays exponentially. This process is known as *inactivation*. It may be described in the kinetic scheme by supposing that one of the gates moves more slowly than others and moves in the *opposite* direction, i.e. it closes on depolarization of the membrane. Hodgkin and Huxley chose the variable m to describe the sodium activation process and the variable h to describe the inactivation process. Three m gates and one h gate were found to

25

Theory of electric current flow in excitable tissues

give the best fit, so that

$$i_{Na^+} = m^3 h \bar{g}_{Na} (\vec{u} - E_{Na^+}), \qquad (2.9)$$

where m and h obey equations similar to eqn (2.5).

Fig. 2.4 shows the way in which eqns (2.8) and (2.9) (together with, of course, appropriate functions for the αs and βs designed to fit experimental results) reproduce the experimentally observed changes in conductance to sodium and potassium ions. Note that in each case an increase in the magnitude of the depolarization not only increases the magnitude of the conductance increase but also the speed of its onset. This is expected since the opening rate coefficient α will increase as the potential is made more positive. Similar behaviour is shown by the currents observed in cardiac muscle (see e.g. Fig. 7.3, p. 93). It is also important to note the time-scale of the events shown in Fig. 2.4. The Na^+ current activates within a millisecond. The onset of the K^+ current and the decay of the Na^+ current occur more slowly but are still complete within 5–10 ms. These time-scales are appropriate to the time-scale of the action potential in squid nerve. Fig. 2.5 shows the action potential

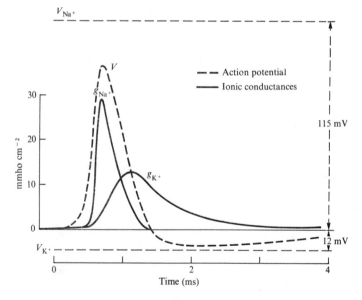

FIG. 2.5. Action potential and ionic conductances given by Hodgkin–Huxley theory of the nerve impulse (Hodgkin and Huxley 1952).

computed by Hodgkin and Huxley, together with the calculated conductance changes. These computations very successfully reproduced
the experimental records of potential and conductance changes in squid
nerve.

Application of theory to cardiac muscle

It is evident from Fig. 1.3 (p. 7) that without some modification,
the Hodgkin—Huxley equations cannot reproduce the action potentials
in cardiac muscle. In the first place, the time-scale is quite different.
Cardiac action potentials are measured in hundreds of milliseconds.
Moreover the shape of the potential change is very different. The repolarization process in cardiac muscle is extremely slow compared to the
depolarization (see Chapter 6), whereas in nerve fibres the two processes
occur at more comparable rates, although depolarization is generally
significantly faster. Finally, as we shall show later (see Chapter 6), the
membrane conductance during the cardiac action potential is very low
once the initial depolarization phase is complete, whereas in nerve the
total conductance ($g_{Na^+} + g_{K^+}$) is elevated throughout the action potential, as first shown experimentally by Cole and Curtis (1939).

Nevertheless, it is interesting to ask whether there are any modifications of the Hodgkin—Huxley equations that will reproduce action
potentials like those observed in cardiac muscle. Theoretical studies in
1960 showed that remarkably simple modifications of the equations
will produce cardiac-like action potentials (FitzHugh 1960; George and
Johnson 1961; Brady and Woodbury 1960; Noble 1960, 1962a). FitzHugh
and George and Johnson showed that reducing the speed and magnitude
of the K^+ conductance is sufficient to produce a plateau in the repolarization phase. Brady and Woodbury showed that including a slow phase
of Na^+ current inactivation has a similar effect. My own calculations
were based on some early experimental measurements of the potassium
conductance changes in cardiac muscle (Hutter and Noble 1960; Hall,
Hutter, and Noble 1963) which showed that in Purkinje fibres the K^+
conductance displayed two components. The first, $g_{K^+, 1}$, is time-
independent and shows the phenomenon of inward-going rectification
discussed earlier in this chapter. The second, $g_{K^+, 2}$, is a small and greatly
slowed time-dependent component obeying Hodgkin—Huxley kinetics,
which is similar to the single K^+ conductance postulated in FitzHugh's
work. These experiments suggested that the effect of depolarization on
the K^+ conductance in cardiac muscle is twofold: first a large fall in

/ inward going rectification ?

conductance (which is *not* observed in normal squid nerve); then a
time-dependent increase (which is much smaller and much slower than
in squid nerve). The calculations were undertaken to determine whether
the incorporation of these experimental results into modified K^+ current
equations would be sufficient to account for the highly characteristic
action potentials and pacemaker activity in cardiac Purkinje fibres.

Fig. 2.6 shows the degree of success that could be obtained with this
approach. The calculated potential changes are remarkably like those
observed experimentally in spontaneously active Purkinje fibres (see
Fig. 1.3 (e), p. 7). The conductance curves plotted below the computed
potential record show how this is achieved. The first phase of depolarization is generated by the activation of the Na^+ conductance as in nerve.
The Na^+ conductance then largely, but not completely, inactivates.
The incompleteness of the inactivation of the Na^+ conductance at some
potentials is an inherent feature of the Hodgkin–Huxley equations (see
Noble 1966). It was not introduced as a modification.

This residual Na^+ conductance is of no consequence in nerve fibres
since the membrane is repolarized by the K^+ current long before the
residual Na^+ conductance can exert an effect. By contrast, in heart,
where the K^+ conductance *falls* at the beginning of depolarization, the
residual Na^+ conductance can help to maintain the depolarization during
the plateau phase.

The plateau phase is terminated as the time-dependent K^+ conductance
$g_{K^+,2}$ activates. Notice also that the computation shown in Fig. 2.6 then
reproduces another important property of cardiac muscle. The decay of
$g_{K^+,2}$ is responsible for generating the pacemaker potential by allowing
the resting Na^+ conductance to depolarize the membrane towards the
threshold for initiating another action potential. Other features of
cardiac muscle that may be reproduced with these equations include
the conductance changes, the effects of variations in firing frequency
and the responses to applied currents (see Noble 1962a).

Nevertheless, the success of this model is partly deceptive. A decade
later, following extensive experimental analyses of the ionic currents
in cardiac membranes using the voltage-clamp technique, we can see both
where the model is incorrect and why it worked as well as it did. The
actual variations in conductance to outward and inward currents in the
Purkinje fibre are not at all dissimilar from those shown in Fig. 2.6, but
the ionic components and the kinetics and other properties of the channels
differ from those used in the 1962 model in striking and fundamental
ways. Unfortunately for students and clinicians, the story has, in the

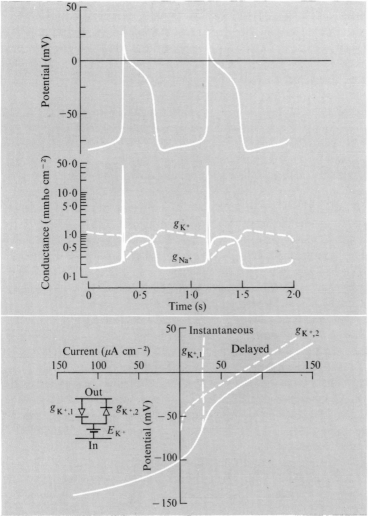

FIG. 2.6. A model of cardiac action potentials and pacemaker activity based on a modification of the Hodgkin–Huxley theory. The Na⁺ current is given by the Hodgkin–Huxley sodium equations with slight modifications to allow enough sodium current to flow to maintain the plateau. The K⁺ conductance $g_{K^+, 1}$ is dependent on voltage only and shows inward-rectification. This component becomes very small when the membrane is depolarized. $g_{K^+, 2}$ is described by the Hodgkin–Huxley K⁺ equations using greatly slowed kinetics. These properties of g_{K^+} were based on results of Hall, Hutter, and Noble (1963). The top record shows the computed potential changes which closely resemble experimental records (see Fig. 1.3(e)). Changes in g_{Na^+} and g_{K^+} are plotted below. The way in which the total K⁺ current is divided into two components is shown in bottom diagram. This model will be referred to as the 1962 model.

process, become considerably more complex. It may help the reader, therefore, to indicate how the various components of ionic current that I shall describe in later chapters may be fitted into a general scheme by explaining how they may serve one or other of the functions served by the conductance changes shown in Fig. 2.6. I shall do this by summarizing the essential features of the conductance changes of the 1962 model and how they might be modified without detracting from the model's ability to reproduce the experimentally observed potential changes.

1. The initial transient conductance increase must be large enough to account for the maximum rate of depolarization observed. Despite the long-lasting nature of the cardiac action potential, the initial rate of depolarization is frequently as large as in nerve fibres (of the order of $500\,mV\,ms^{-1}$, i.e. an upstroke time of less than a millisecond to depolarize the membrane by rather more than 100 mV). Although this point is not clear in Fig. 2.6, the 1962 model did not achieve this high rate of depolarization without supposing that only part of the cell membrane is depolarized by the initial conductance change (Noble 1962b). I shall discuss this problem in Chapter 4, where we shall find that the problem is still with us and is still not fully resolved.

2. The residual conductance to inward-moving ions must be large enough to maintain the depolarization during the plateau. However, it is clearly not essential that this conductance should be controlled by the same gating mechanisms as those responsible for the time course of the initial Na^+ conductance. In fact, it is now known that a substantial part of the inward current flowing during the action potential plateau is carried by calcium ions and that a completely separate gating mechanism is involved. This is one of the most important discoveries made using the voltage-clamp technique in cardiac muscle and I shall discuss it, and its relevance to the initiation of contraction, in Chapter 5.

3. In the 1962 model, the initial fall in g_{K^+} was restricted to $g_{K^+,1}$. The time-dependent component of K^+ conductance was not assumed to show inward-going rectification. Indeed, at that time, it would have appeared unnecessarily complicated to suppose that channels gated by Hodgkin—Huxley mechanisms could also show the curious behaviour of inward-rectification. Nevertheless, there is nothing inherent in the modelling that requires this rectification to be restricted to $g_{K^+,1}$. Indeed, the maintainance of the plateau would require an even smaller inward current if the time-dependent K^+ conductance were to respond to sudden depolarization with a reduction in permeability. In Chapter 7, I shall show that the K^+ conductance $g_{K^+,2}$ responsible for pacemaker activity

in Purkinje fibres does show this rather bizarre combination of properties.

4. Termination of the action potential, i.e. repolarization, may be attributed to a slow increase in K^+ conductance, as in Fig. 2.6 but it might equally well be attributed to a slow fall in conductance to an inward-moving ion, as postulated by Brady and Woodbury (1960). The mechanisms of repolarization are important clinically as well as physiologically, and I shall discuss them at some length in Chapter 6. It will be shown that *both* types of conductance change contribute to repolarization, although to varying degrees in different parts of the heart.

5. The decay of K^+ conductance responsible for pacemaker activity need not involve the same mechanism as that contributing to the termination of the plateau. In 1962, given the object of discovering how *simple* modifications of the Hodgkin–Huxley equations would work, and given the paucity of experimental information on the K^+ conductance beyond that of Hall, Hutter, and Noble (1963), it would have been perverse to postulate the existence of more than one time-dependent K^+ conductance. Today, we are forced by the experimental data to recognize the existence of several time-dependent K^+ conductances, none of which possesses kinetics appropriate to determining both repolarization *and* pacemaker activity in Purkinje fibres. The experiments that have led to this result will be discussed in Chapter 7.

6. Finally and most importantly it must be emphasized that, as Fig. 1.3 shows, there are substantial variations in the electrical behaviour of different parts of the heart and these must be reflected in the underlying ionic current mechanisms. The most striking example of these differences that I shall discuss concerns pacemaker mechanisms. In Chapter 7 I shall show that the atrial and Purkinje fibre pacemaker mechanisms are sign-ʿ ʿantly different, despite the fact that they are both controlled by K^+ conductance decays. In Chapter 8 I shall discuss the even more striking fact that this difference is reflected in the quite different mechanisms by which adrenaline accelerates the two kinds of pacemaker.

A note on cable theory and its application to cardiac muscle

Few areas of electrophysiology are more likely, by virtue of their inherent difficulty, to deter medical students than the theory of current spread along excitable cells. Therefore I have deliberately placed this section at the end of the chapter. The reader who wishes to omit the more mathematical aspects of excitation and conduction may skip this section and move on to subsequent chapters. However, the subject cannot be entirely neglected in a book of this nature. The interpretation of voltage-clamp records often requires a good knowledge of cable theory despite the fact that a *perfect* voltage-clamp experiment eliminates the cable problems. The trouble is that few voltage-clamp experiments are perfect (indeed in heart muscle I think we can safely say that none are). Moreover, the phenomenon of conduction, which is important in the heart, cannot be treated without cable theory. I shall therefore give a brief account. The more serious student is referred to the book by Jack, Noble, and Tsien (1975) which gives a more advanced treatment of the physics and mathematics of excitation and conduction.

The propagation of the impulse depends on the flow of electric current along the muscle fibres from active to resting regions of the heart. In some regions (e.g. the Purkinje fibres) this process involves flow along a cylindrical fibre and only one spatial dimension is involved. In most regions of the heart the spread occurs in a more complex geometrical network as the impulse spreads over and through the walls of the atria and ventricles. The theory of multidimensional spread of current is more complex (see Jack, Noble, and Tsien (1975), Chapters 5 and 7) and in this account I shall consider only the spread in a cylindrical fibre

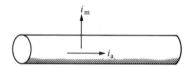

FIG. 2.7. Cable model of excitable cell. The axial current is i_a, the current crossing the membrane is i_m. Any change in i_a must therefore reflect the flow of i_m.

(see Fig. 2.7). The axial flow of current in the myoplasm is i_a. The membrane current is i_m. We shall assume the fibre to be immersed in a very large volume of extracellular fluid so that extracellular potentials may be negligibly small.

If the intracellular phase (myoplasm) acts as a simple resistance the flow of current along it will be proportional to the voltage gradient (Ohm's law). Hence

$$\frac{\partial V}{\partial x} = -r_a i_a, \tag{2.10}$$

where r_a is the myoplasm resistance per unit length of fibre.

The question whether the intracellular phase in cardiac muscle acts as a simple resistance has been a controversial one. Unlike nerve or skeletal muscle fibres, cardiac muscle fibres are not composed of single cylinders. Each fibre is composed of a large number of closely apposed cells, each of which is surrounded by a complete envelope of membrane. This anatomical feature led some people to propose that conduction between cardiac cells does not occur by a simple flow of electric current and that there might be a chemical intermediate, as in transmission at the neuromuscular junction. However, although the membrane around each cardiac cell is complete, there are regions (the nexuses) at which the membranes come into very close contact. The structure of these contact regions suggests that they are specialized to allow conduction of ions and other small molecules between the cells (see review by McNutt and Weinstein (1973)).

The physiological evidence certainly suggests that this is the case. Fig. 2.8 shows the result of an important experiment by Barr, Dewey, and Berger to test whether conduction occurs as the result of the flow of i_a between cardiac cells. As we have already noted in discussing the electrocardiogram in Chapter 1, the intra and extracellular fluids form parts of a closed circuit during propagation. Hence, if we interrupt the extracellular flow of current by a high resistance, we should prevent the flow of i_a and so prevent propagation. Barr, Dewey, and Berger (1965) achieved this by allowing a strip of heart muscle to pass through a sucrose gap (see p. 42). The sucrose solution contains very few ions and so has a high resistance. They then determined whether the action potential initiated on one side of the gap would spread to the other side. This is simple to detect by recording the potential across the gap, the action potential on one side will be positive and that on the other side will be negative. A monophasic record will therefore indicate the absence of conduction while a diphasic record indicates that conduction has occurred.[†]

The result is clear: the record is monophasic when the gap resistance is high. The high-resistance sucrose gap therefore blocks conduction which must depend on local circuit current flow. This may be further tested by shorting the sucrose resistance with lower resistances placed in parallel. A low enough resistance allows sufficient local circuit current to flow again and conduction (indicated by a diphasic record) returns. The action potentials recorded are then smaller since the resistance across which they are recorded is smaller.

[†] As shown in Fig. 1.3 (p. 7), single action potentials are monophasic. Hence a diphasic record can only be formed by algebraic summation of two action potentials of opposite sign, with one of the action potentials displaced in time by the time taken for conduction to occur across the gap.

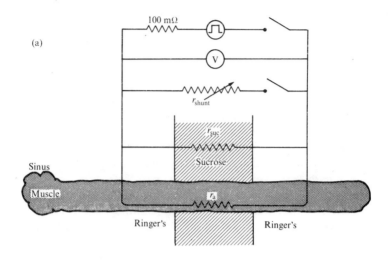

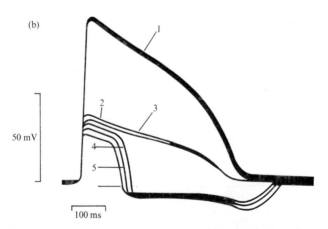

FIG. 2.8. Experimental test of theory of electric conduction in cardiac muscle (frog atrial muscle). (a) Experimental arrangement. One end of muscle strip is isolated from the other by high-resistance sucrose gap, across which the voltage could be recorded and shunt resistances were placed. The preparation is excited by applying a brief pulse to a 100 MΩ resistor. (b) Records of action potentials. Curves 1–6 are obtained with shunt resistance of ∞, 10^5, 9×10^4, 8×10^4, 7×10^4, and 6×10^4 Ω respectively. Width of sucrose gap is 500 μm. Conduction across the gap is indicated by diphasic wave when shunt resistance is less than 9×10^4 Ω (records 4, 5, and 6) (Barr, Dewey, and Berger 1965).

Weidmann (1966) provided evidence of a different kind. He showed that radioactive potassium ions will diffuse along cardiac fibres from cell to cell to a degree that requires fairly free diffusion across the cell contacts. He had also earlier (Weidmann 1952) provided evidence, using cable theory, that electric current flows freely between Purkinje fibre cells. An excellent account of cell-to-cell conduction in cardiac muscle is given in Weidmann's *Harvey Lecture* (Weidmann 1967).

For most practical purposes, therefore, we may represent the intracellular medium, including the cell-to-cell contacts, by the resistance r_a. However, careful measurements of the electrical properties of Purkinje fibres have shown that the capacitative coupling between cells that may also be expected at regions of close apposition is also present (Freygang and Trautwein 1970).

As the axial current flows along a fibre, some of it leaks across the surface membrane as membrane current. The amount of membrane current in any region therefore must be equal and opposite to the *change* in axial current across the region. Thus

$$i_m = -\partial i_a / \partial x. \tag{2.11}$$

Eqns (2.10) and (2.11) give us two equations containing i_a. To combine them we differentiate eqn (2.10) to allow the term $\partial i_a / \partial x$ to be eliminated:

$$\frac{\partial^2 V}{\partial x^2} = -r_a \frac{\partial i_a}{\partial x} = r_a i_m. \tag{2.12}$$

This gives us the important result that the total membrane current is proportional to the second derivative of the voltage. It should be emphasized, however, that i_m is the *total* membrane current. This includes the ionic current discussed earlier in this chapter but it also includes a component that I have not yet discussed but which is very important in determining the speed of the potential changes produced by the ionic currents. This component is the capacity current flow i_c. The nature of this current is often puzzling to medical students and, in view of its importance in excitation phenomena in the heart, I think it is worth explaining the membrane capacity and the capacity current in a little detail.

The membrane is a thin layer formed of phospholipids and proteins. The evidence from physical studies (see Levine 1972) shows that the hydrophobic (oily) parts of the molecules (i.e. the fatty-acid chains of the phospholipids and the non-polar parts of the proteins) are arranged to form an inner layer of low dielectric constant about 50 Å in thickness.

This layer lies between the hydrophilic layers formed by the phospholipid headgroups. These layers, and the highly conducting salt solutions on either side of the membrane, are polar and have high dielectric constants. This arrangement is equivalent to that of a parallel-plate condenser, the solutions corresponding to the conducting plates and the hydrophobic layer to the low dielectric medium separating the plates.

When a current i_c is applied to a condenser, charge $(i_c \times t)$ is added to one plate and subtracted from the other. Thus a potential difference develops. This potential is proportional to the charge Q applied,

$$Q = cV = i_c t, \tag{2.13}$$

where c is the capacitance of the condenser (i.e. the amount of charge it will accumulate to produce a unit voltage).

The value of c depends on the thickness and dielectric constant of the layer between the plates. A large capacitance is obtained when the layer is thin and the dielectric constant is low. These are the conditions that occur in biological membranes. It is not surprising therefore that they show a relatively high capacitance (about $1 \ \mu F \ cm^{-2}$). The significance of this capacitance may be shown by calculating how it determines the rate of potential change produced by currents similar to those developed in cardiac cells. The equation for the speed of voltage change is obtained by differentiating eqn (2.13):

$$c \frac{dV}{dt} = i_c. \tag{2.14}$$

Thus, to depolarize a cell membrane at a rate of $500 \ mV \ ms^{-1}$ (see p. 30 above) we require, since $500 \ mV \ ms^{-1} = 500 \ V \ s^{-1}$,

$$1 \times 10^{-6} \ F \times 500 \ V \ s^{-1} = 500 \ \mu A. \tag{2.15}$$

As we shall see later (Chapter 4) this current is very large compared to the Na^+ currents recorded experimentally in cardiac muscle. I shall discuss the problems created by this discrepancy in that chapter.

As noted already, the repolarization rate in cardiac muscle is very slow, and is usually less than $1 \ mV \ ms^{-1}$. We then require only

$$1 \times 10^{-6} F \times 1 \ V \ s^{-1} = 1 \ \mu A. \tag{2.16}$$

I shall discuss the factors determining the repolarization rate in Chapter 6.

The total membrane current i_m is given by the sum of the capacitance and ionic currents,

$$i_m = i_c + i_i = c\frac{\partial V}{\partial t} + i_i. \tag{2.17}$$

This equation may be visualized by regarding i_c as the current that provides the charge that accumulates on the membrane capacitance while i_i is the charge that leaks through the membrane channels.

When an action potential is initiated in a small isolated segment of muscle in which the potential changes are uniform (i.e. there is no propagation), all the charge that moves through the membrane channels is used to change the charge on the local membrane capacitance. There is no net current flow into or away from the cell, i_m is zero, and i_c is equal and opposite to i_i. We then have the equation for a *uniform* (sometimes called m*embrane*) action potential:

$$dV/dt = -i_i/c. \tag{2.18}$$

During propagation, the situation is more complex and net membrane current does flow as charge moves from one cell to the next. As already shown, the total membrane current is then given by eqn (2.12). Combining eqns (2.12) and (2.17) we obtain

$$\frac{1}{r_a}\frac{\partial^2 V}{\partial x^2} = c\frac{\partial V}{\partial t} + i_i \tag{2.19}$$

There is one situation for which this equation may be greatly simplified. During steady propagation the action potential moves along the fibre at a constant conduction velocity θ, so that in time t a distance θt is travelled. The action potential waveform therefore has the same shape whether plotted as a function of x or of θt. This point has already been noted in Chapter 1 (eqn (1.2)). Using eqn (1.2) to simplify eqn (2.19) we obtain

$$\frac{1}{r_a\theta^2}\frac{d^2 V}{dt^2} = c\frac{dV}{dt} + i_i. \tag{2.20}$$

This equation implicitly defines the conduction velocity in terms of the ionic current flow, the membrane capacitance, the axial resistance. All these parameters depend on the size of the fibre. The axial resistance decreases as the cross-sectional area πr^2 of the fibre increases. Hence r_a will be related to the specific resistivity R_i of the intracellular fluid by

$$r_a = R_i/\pi r^2. \tag{2.21}$$

By contrast, the capacitance and ionic current scale vary as the membrane area which varies as the circumference $2\pi r$. Hence

$$i_i = 2\pi r I_i, \tag{2.22}$$

$$c = 2\pi r C, \tag{2.23}$$

where I_i and C are the ionic current and capacitance per unit area of membrane. If the specific properties of the components do not vary with fibre size R_i, C, and I_i will be independent of r. Using (2.21), (2.22), and (2.23), eqn (2.20) becomes

$$\frac{r}{2R_i\theta^2}\frac{\mathrm{d}^2V}{\mathrm{d}t^2} = C\frac{\mathrm{d}V}{\mathrm{d}t} + I_i. \tag{2.24}$$

All terms in the equation apart from θ and r itself are now independent of r. Hence r/θ^2 must also be independent of r, so that we must have

$$\theta \propto \sqrt{r}, \tag{2.25}$$

which gives the familiar result that the conduction velocity is largest in large fibres.

The speed of transmission is an important factor in cardiac excitation since it is the function of the conducting system to ensure that the mechanical events are correctly timed (Chapter 1, p. 4). The conduction velocity is very low (about $0.2\ \mathrm{ms}^{-1}$) in the AV node to ensure a significant delay between auricular and ventricular contraction. By contrast the impulse travels very rapidly (about $4\ \mathrm{ms}^{-1}$) in the Purkinje fibres to ensure nearly synchronous excitation of the ventricle. As expected, the fibres of the AV node are very small (about $7\ \mu\mathrm{m}$ in radius), whereas those of the Purkinje fibre system are large (about $50\ \mu\mathrm{m}$ in radius).

However, fibre diameter is not the only important factor. The excitatory ionic current generated by the cells of the AV node is much smaller than that generated by the Purkinje fibres. This further increases the difference between their conduction velocities, which is clearly larger than expected from the difference in fibre diameters ($\sqrt{(50/7)}$ is only 2.7, compared to a ratio of conduction velocities of $4/0.2 = 20$). Under some circumstances, the excitatory ionic current generated by Purkinje fibres may also become small. The consequences of this situation for the functioning of the heart will be discussed in Chapter 10.

3 Methods for studying ionic currents in cardiac muscle

The potential changes in cardiac cells are determined by the ionic currents flowing across the cell membranes. The ionic currents in turn, are determined by the changes in membrane potential, as discussed in Chapter 2. To measure the ionic currents it is therefore necessary to control the membrane potential. This was first achieved in nerve axons by Cole (1949) and Marmont (1949) using the giant nerve fibres of the squid. The object of their technique (usually called the voltage-clamp technique) is to control the membrane potential by holding ('clamping') it at values chosen by the experimenter and keeping it uniform over an area of membrane through which the recorded current flows. In squid nerve, uniformity of potential was achieved by inserting a wire electrode along the axoplasm. The axoplasm resistance r_a was thus shorted and the membrane of the nerve could be polarized uniformly.

This technique is not applicable to cardiac muscle fibres which are far too small to allow wire electrodes to be inserted. Uniformity of current flow and potential must therefore be achieved in other ways. Two basic techniques have been developed: microelectrode techniques and sucrose-gap techniques. A third technique is a hybrid one using a combination of microelectrode recording and sucrose gaps.

Two microelectrode techniques

To control the membrane potential one must be able to pass current across the cell membrane. One way of doing this is to apply currents using a fine glass microelectrode inserted inside the cell. A second microelectrode is also inserted to record the membrane potential. By inserting the electrodes close together the potential may be recorded at the site of current injection. This technique was used in the early 1950s (see e.g. Weidmann 1951) to measure membrane resistances in cardiac cells, and some of the important results will be discussed in Chapter 6. The current however not only flows through the membrane of the cell into which the electrodes are inserted. It also flows along the axial resistance to other cells. As it does so, some current flows through the membranes of adjacent cells and so the current (and the potential produced) decays as a function of distance from the site of current injection. The rate of the decay is determined by the ratio r_m/r_a since the relative ease with which current crosses the cell membrane compared to flowing along the axial resistance determines the extent of spatial spread. A large value of r_m keeps the current leak through the membranes low, and a low value of r_a helps it to flow along the fibre. When the appropriate cable equations (see p. 45 at the end of this chapter) are solved, the constant $\sqrt{(r_m/r_a)}$ is found to give the distance required for the voltage to decay to approximately one third of its value at the site of current injection. This constant is called the *space-constant* λ. Thus, in Purkinje fibres, λ is 2 mm (Weidmann 1952). A fibre only 4—5 millimetres long will therefore be very non-uniformly polarized.

Deck, Kern, and Trautwein (1964) were the first to make use of the fact that cut or otherwise damaged cardiac muscle 'heals over', the result being a high resistance seal at or near the site of the damage or cut (Weidmann 1967; Délèze 1970). By using this property, it is possible to isolate a small segment (e.g. 1 mm) of a Purkinje fibre and to insert two glass microelectrodes. By placing the electrodes in the centre of the segment, the end of the fibre may be only 0·5 mm or 0·25λ away from the electrode. Even in a segment as long as 2 mm, the end is only 0·5λ away. Under these conditions, the non-uniformity of voltage produced by passing current at the centre of the fibre may be restricted to within 5—10 per cent (see Jack, Noble, and Tsien (1975), Chapter 4, for a theoretical treatment of this kind of problem in cable theory).

Of course, this estimate applies strictly only when the space-constant remains as long as 2 mm. This condition requires that the membrane resistance r_m should remain high (or that the membrane conductance $1/r_m$ should remain small). In studies of the K^+ conductance, this is usually the case over at least some ranges of potential. As we have seen in Chapter 2 (p. 27) the initial effect of membrane depolarization is to reduce the K^+ conductance so that the effective space constant becomes larger than normal. Provided that the subsequent recovery of conductance is not too great one may expect the uniformity of polarization to be maintained. Deck, Kern, and Trautwein (1964) checked this point experimentally by inserting a third microelectrode so that they could measure the membrane potential at two different points. Very little difference in potential was observed.

However, the situation is not as encouraging as this when the Na^+ currents are investigated. As shown in Chapter 2 (p. 30), the Na^+ conductance undergoes a very large increase on depolarization. The question whether the membrane may be controlled adequately during this time is more problematic and I shall return to this point in Chapter 4.

In addition to ensuring that the membrane potential is uniform in the region being studied, the voltage-clamp technique also requires that the potential should be controlled, usually by being made to follow a step-waveform from one constant potential to another. The introduction of electronic circuits to achieve this is quite a complex matter and the details vary greatly between one laboratory and another. However, the principle involved is very simple and is illustrated in Fig. 3.1.

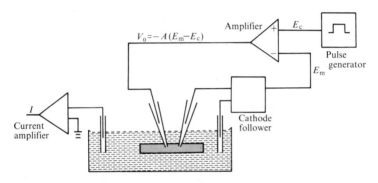

FIG. 3.1. General arrangement of circuit for voltage-clamp work. The membrane potential E_m of a short Purkinje fibre is recorded with a microelectrode and, after passing through a cathode follower to prevent significant current being drawn from the fibre, is fed to the negative input of an amplifier that amplifies the signal by a factor $-A$. The voltage-clamp signal E_c is fed into the positive input. The output $-A(E_m - E_c)$ is applied to interior of fibre via a second microelectrode. Current flowing through membrane is collected by an electrode connected to a current amplifier.

In all cases, use is made of an amplifier whose inputs are the membrane potential E_m and a command potential E_c generated by a square-wave generator. The output is the difference between these potentials amplified by a factor A. The output is opposite in sign to the membrane potential, which is therefore multiplied by $-A$. The command potential is applied to a 'positive' input and is multiplied by A. The output is therefore proportional to $-A(E_m - E_c)$. This voltage is applied to the current electrode. We may now show that this has the effect of making E_m follow E_c. Suppose that E_m is initially -80 mV and E_c is suddenly switched to 0. $E_m - E_c$ is therefore equal to -80 mV. The output voltage

will be positive, i.e. $80A$ mV. A positive (depolarizing) current is therefore applied to the current electrode which therefore depolarizes the
membrane. The magnitude of the depolarizing current will only diminish
as E_m approaches E_c. If the amplification factor A is sufficiently large,
the effect is that E_m is forced to closely follow E_c. In theory, by making
A as large as we wish, we can force E_m to follow E_c as closely as we
please. In practice, however, there are technical limits on the magnitude
of A. When microelectrodes are used these arise from the limitations
on the amount of current that may flow through the large resistance
provided by the current electrode, and from the fact that two electrodes
placed close together may pass current directly between each other at
high frequencies by virtue of the capacitance between them. These
technical problems can lead to unstable oscillatory behaviour at large
values of A. It is usually necessary therefore to keep A below a certain
value and allow a small ($1-2$ mV) difference between E_m and E_c to
remain.

Double sucrose-gap technique

The use of a sucrose gap to isolate the extracellular phases of two
regions of heart muscle has already been discussed in Chapter 2 (Fig.
2.8, p. 34) in describing the experiment on conduction by Barr, Dewey,
and Berger. Rougier, Vassort, and Stämpfli (1968) developed this approach
to allow voltage-clamp experiments to be performed. The principle is that
the external resistance between two or more regions of the fibre is greatly
increased by replacing the normal salt solutions bathing the tissue by an
ion-deficient sucrose solution (the sucrose is included simply to maintain
the osmotic pressure). The result is that the regions on each side of a gap
are effectively connected via only the intracellular phase. If current is
applied between the two regions it will flow into the cells in one region,
and along the intracellular fluid (passing from cell to cell via the intercellular connections) to pass out through the cell membranes of the other
region. The technique may therefore be used to apply current intracellularly without using microelectrodes. As I have already noted in Chapter
2, the method may also be used to record the membrane potential. More
strictly, the technique measures the difference between the potentials of
the two regions. If one region is kept at constant potential, the extracellular potential across the gap will follow the intracellular potential of
the region whose potential is varying.

Fig. 3.2 shows how the technique is applied to cardiac muscle. A fine
strip of tissue, typically 100 μm or less in diameter and a few millimetres

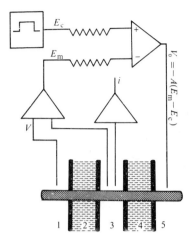

FIG. 3.2. Diagram of bath and circuit used in voltage-clamp experiments on atrial muscle. Chambers 2 and 4 are perfused with sucrose. Chamber 1 is used to record the potential changes with respect to the test gap (3). Chamber 5 is used to apply current flow to test gap.

in length, is dissected from the heart. The most suitable preparations are obtained from amphibian atria where the inner wall is lined with fine trabeculae of the right dimensions and requiring relatively little cutting from the wall. With care it is possible to isolate relatively long intact trabeculae. The trabeculum is then placed in a bath so that it runs across five chambers. The length of the preparation in the middle 'test' region is kept very small (e.g. 100–400 μm) and is exposed to physiological solutions. The chambers on either side are filled with sucrose solution. The end chambers are filled with a physiological solution which may be K^+-rich to depolarize the ends of the preparation. The potential difference between one of the end chambers and the middle chamber then gives a measure of the membrane potential of the cells in the middle 'test' chamber.

There are several variations on the technique. Some techniques dispense with both partitions and rely simply on streamlined flow of the ion and sucrose solutions to create separate regions. This technique has the advantage that the dimensions of the test region under voltage control may be varied in attempts to find an optimum length (see e.g. Hemptinne 1973).

The success of the current application, and even more of the voltage recording, depends on the resistance of the interior of the preparation being negligible compared to the external resistance of the sucrose gap.

43

This may be tested by recording the action potentials and resting potentials using the sucrose-gap technique and comparing them with those recorded using intracellular microelectrodes. Fig. 3.3 shows such a test.

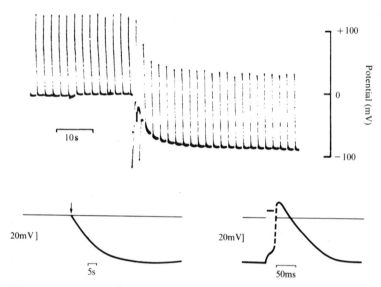

FIG. 3.3. Measurement of resting and action potentials of atrial muscle using sucrose-gap technique. Top record shows development of 'resting potential' during application of isotonic KCl solution to chamber 1 (see Fig. 3.2) while chamber 3 (the test gap) is perfused with normal Ringer solution. Tracing shows pen recordings of action potentials in response to repetitive stimuli applied via chamber 5. Note presence of two 'inverted action potentials' arising in chamber 1 immediately following application of K$^+$ solution. The resting potential in this case is -80 mV and the action-potential overshoot is $+30$ mV (Brown and Noble 1969a). Bottom record shows an alternative method. The test gap is first depolarized in isotonic K$^+$ solution and the recovery of potential is then observed following return to normal Ringer (left). The action potential (right) is similar to that recorded using intracellular electrodes (see Fig. 1.3(b)) (Ojeda 1971).

The resting potential (-80 mV) and action potential (120 mV) are as large as those recorded with intracellular microelectrodes. Virtually all the voltage drop must therefore occur in the external sucrose gap across which the voltage is recorded while negligibly small voltage drops occur within the preparation. Since an identical gap is also used for applying current, this also ensures that very little of the current applied at one of the ends flows through the external resistance of the gap. Most of it must flow through the interior of the fibres and then across the membrane in the central test gap.

Voltage-clamp conditions in the test gap are then achieved using circuits like that illustrated in Fig. 3.1. The two microelectrodes are simply replaced by metal electrodes lying in the end chambers.

Hybrid techniques

It is also possible to use a sucrose gap to apply current to a region whose membrane potential is recorded with a microelectrode. This hybrid method is most frequently used in work on ventricular muscle (Beeler and Reuter 1970*a*; Giebisch and Weidmann 1972; New and Trautwein 1972*a*). There are two major advantages. First, in some cases the sucrose gap may not have a high enough resistance to record the membrane potential effectively. Provided the membrane potential is recorded accurately with a microelectrode, the sucrose gap may still be used to apply current. The 'leak' current in this case will be larger, which makes it difficult or impossible accurately to record currents that do not vary with time (see p. 119).

Second, if the test region is free at one end it may be attached to a tension recorder to record mechanical events at the same time as applying a voltage clamp to the muscle. This technique has been invaluable in work on the link between electrical and mechanical events (see Chapter 5).

Problems in achieving spatial uniformity

As in the previous chapter, I have left the more difficult and mathematical aspects of the subject to the end to be omitted if desired. It would however be misleading not to give some words of warning on the use and interpretation of voltage-clamp experiments in cardiac muscle. Some workers have questioned whether any of the results are interpretable and it is virtually agreed that the results should be interpreted with great care. The possible sources of errors and artefacts are several and it may not be possible to eliminate or control all of them. The best we can hope for is a compromise, and that the results of different methods may be compared to control for all but common errors.

Spatial non-uniformity may arise in at least three different ways. First, the length of the fibre being clamped is important. The steady-state distribution of potential along the fibre is given by eqn (2.12) with i_m set to V/r_m, which gives on rearranging:

$$d^2V/dx^2 = V/\lambda^2, \qquad (3.1)$$

$$\frac{dV^2}{dx^2} = -r_a \frac{di_a}{dx} = r_a i_m$$

where $\lambda = \sqrt{(r_m/r_a)}$. A solution to this equation is

$$V = Ae^{-x/\lambda} + Be^{x/\lambda}, \tag{3.2}$$

where A and B are constants. For a cable of infinite length, B must be zero since V must decline towards zero a long way from the current source ($e^{x/\lambda}$ increases with distance and must therefore be eliminated). We then obtain

$$V = V_0 e^{-x/\lambda}, \tag{3.3}$$

where A is given by the voltage V_0 at $x = 0$. This equation describes an exponential decay of voltage with distance and, as noted earlier in the chapter, V falls to about a third of its initial value in one space constant. When the fibre is not very long, the constant B may not be eliminated and the positive exponential term adds to the negative one. This ensures that the presence of a high resistance (either of a healed end or of a sucrose gap) at the end of the fibre decreases the rate of decay of potential. Thus, in a fibre one space-constant long the potential falls to 66 per cent instead of to 37 per cent. At shorter lengths the effect is even more dramatic (see Jack, Noble and Tsien (1975), Chapter 4) and a fibre half a space-constant in length is uniform to within 10 per cent. This is the theoretical basis of using short segments to achieve relative uniformity. As already noted above, non-uniformitities will arise as soon as the space-constant falls to a small enough value. I shall discuss a case of this kind in the next chapter (p. 56).

Secondly, it is important to remember that a cardiac muscle fibre is a tightly packed bundle of cells with narrow clefts between the cells (Sommer and Johnson 1968). The resistance of the extracellular fluid in these clefts is large and the extracellular potentials developed in them may be large enough to interfere with the control of the membrane potential (Beeler and Reuter 1970a; Johnson and Lieberman 1971). This is illustrated in Fig. 3.4. The membrane current i_m from the cells deep in the clefts must flow through the cleft resistance r_c before reaching the recording electrode. The potential across this resistance will be $i_m r_c$. Now the potential that is controlled by the clamp circuit is the one that is recorded with respect to the bulk extracellular fluids. This must therefore include the cleft potential. The recorded potential V will therefore be

$$V = E_m + i_m r_c. \tag{3.4}$$

Hence, when i_m is large, as during the intense flow of Na^+ current, V will

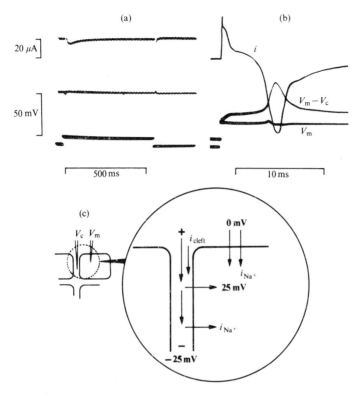

FIG. 3.4. An experiment illustrating the difficulties in achieving uniform potentials during the flow of Na⁺ current. (a) Potential difference (middle trace) between 2 internal microelectrodes during the flow of a relatively small inward Ca^{2+} current (top trace). Note absence of any significant potential difference. The holding potential was set at -40 mV to inactivate g_{Na^+} (see p. 58). (b) Potential difference between one microelectrode in extracellular space within fibre bundle, and one in fibre interior (middle trace) during activation of large Na⁺ current (top trace). Holding potential -80 mV. Note large positive potential develops on extracellular space electrode during flow of inward Na⁺ current. (c) Diagram of situation corresponding to record B. (Beeler and Reuter 1970a.)

differ from E_m by a large amount. Moreover, this difference will be a function of time, since the Na⁺ current varies with time. Since V is held constant by the clamp, E_m must vary and the cells in the interior of the fibre will not be effectively clamped. As shown in Fig. 3.4, the flow of negative (inward) current will require that E_m becomes more positive than V. Beeler and Reuter (1970a) tested this possibility by inserting a microelectrode in the deep extracellular space of a ventricular bundle as

47

well as inserting one intracellularly. They could then record the potential E_m with respect to the immediate extracellular space (thus excluding the cleft potential) as well as the potential V with respect to the bulk extracellular space. The result, as expected, is a large positive variation in the true membrane potential during the flow of the Na^+ current.

Unfortunately, this problem cannot be avoided by using an extracellular cleft electrode in the voltage-clamp circuit since to force the deep cells to follow a step voltage clamp would then produce a negative deviation in the surface cells which are not in series with a significant cleft resistance. The essential problem created by the cleft resistance is therefore one of non-uniformity, and no solution has yet been found for this problem.

Finally, it should be noted that some non-uniformity will be generated in the boundary regions between the ion and sucrose solutions. Diffusion of ions into the sucrose and vice versa will ensure that these boundaries are not sharp and some regions of the test strip will be exposed to solutions with abnormal ion concentrations. This problem becomes most severe when the test gap is short since the diffuse boundary regions then form a larger proportion of the total volume of tissue in the test gap. Hence in seeking an optimum situation at least two opposing factors must be taken into account. The diffuse boundary problem will be most severe in short test gaps while the non-uniformity problem will be most severe in long test gaps.

I shall discuss these problems further when the ionic currents recorded in cardiac muscle are described in subsequent chapters.

4 Sodium current and the spread of excitation

The upstroke (depolarization phase) of the action potential in most excitable cells is generated by an inflow of sodium ions (Hodgkin and Katz 1949a; Hodgkin 1951). Experiments on heart muscle before the development of the voltage-clamp technique showed that this is also the case in Purkinje fibres (Draper and Weidmann 1951) and that the gating mechanisms controlling the inactivation of the Na^+ current resemble those found in nerve membranes (Weidmann 1955). Evidence that sodium ions are responsible for depolarization in other parts of the heart was also obtained, although the situation was not entirely clear in view of some reports that excitation can also sometimes occur in Na^+-free solutions (see review by Brady 1964). As we shall show in the next chapter, calcium ions are also capable of carrying sufficient current under some circumstances, so that cardiac action potentials may be obtained in Na^+-free solutions. Indeed in some parts of the heart (e.g. the AV node) the 'calcium' channels may be very important in normal conduction. Nevertheless, there can be little doubt that in normal atrial, Purkinje, and ventricular fibres, the first ionic current recorded on depolarizing the membrane beyond threshold is a Na^+ current similar in time-course to that recorded in nerve fibres. This current follows closely on the decay of the initial capacity current and it is usually impossible to completely separate the two. The nature of the capacity and of the capacity current are also important in determining how quickly the Na^+ current can depolarize the membrane during normal electrical activity (see Chapter 2, p. 36). In turn this depolarization rate determines the speed at which the excitation spreads through the heart. The problems of capacitance, Na^+ current, and propagation are therefore best dealt with together.

Separation of capacitance and Na^+ currents

We have already seen in Chapter 3 that one reason for using voltage-clamp techniques is to control the variable – the membrane potential – that determines the ionic current flow. There is however a second reason: to separate the capacitance and ionic currents. This is achieved by changing the membrane potential from one value to another very quickly. Since the charge on the membrane capacitance changes only when the voltage is changing (i_c is proportional to dV/dt — see p. 36), the capacity current is restricted to an intense surge during the rapid voltage change and should become zero when the voltage is constant. The currents then recorded should be attributable entirely to ion-transfer through the membrane. Thus, in squid nerve, the capacity current lasts for only about 20 μs, which is fairly small compared to the time required to activate the Na^+ conductance (about 200 μs).

In cardiac muscle, the capacity surge at the beginning of a depolarizing step lasts for a much longer period. Thus, in the record from ventricular muscle shown in Fig. 3.4 (p. 47), the capacitance current lasts for nearly 2 ms, which is much longer than the time taken to change the clamp potential. Similar time-courses for the capacity current are found in Purkinje fibres (Fozzard 1966). These results mean that some capacity current continues to flow when the surface membrane potential is constant. This suggests that the potential step cannot occur as quickly across cell membranes deep inside the fibre. Since the deep cell membrane capacitances must be charged or discharged through the high resistance of the clefts already discussed in Chapter 3, they will be charged more slowly, just as a water tank fills more slowly through a high-resistance narrow pipe than through a low-resistance wide pipe. To a first approximation, therefore, the total membrane capacitance may be divided into two components: the surface component C_s which charges quickly and a deep component C_d which charges slowly. Fozzard's (1966) measurements on Purkinje fibres showed that the total capacitance is around 10 μF cm^{-2}, where C_s is about 2·5 μF cm^{-2}, and C_d about 7·5 μF cm^{-2}. Similar estimates have been obtained by Freygang and Trautwein (1970) and by Carmeliet and Willems (1971). The figure for C_s is also similar to that used by Noble (1962b) to compute realistic values for the conduction velocity and the maximum rate of depolarization. This correspondence suggests a possible functional significance of the division into two components. It is likely that C_s is the component that is involved in determining the conduction velocity.

These figures also correspond well with studies on the microstructure of the Purkinje fibre. Mobley and Page (1972) have shown that about 90 per cent of the total cell-membrane area is located in the clefts of the Purkinje fibre. This means that the total membrane area is 10 times larger than the fibre surface area. Since the total capacitance (referred to surface area) is 10 μF cm^{-2}, the true membrane capacitance must be about 1 $\mu F\ cm^{-2}$, which is similar to the value for nerve membranes. The capacitance of the membrane actually at the surface of the fibre will be only about 1 $\mu F\ cm^{-2}$, compared to 2·5 $\mu F\ cm^{-2}$ for C_s quoted above. This discrepancy is not unexpected since areas of cell membrane lining the clefts but lying fairly close to the surface will have only small cleft resistances in series with them. Some at least of the superficial cleft membranes are undoubtedly included in the 'fast' component C_s.

Kinetics of the Na⁺ conductance

Although it is certain that the first time-dependent ionic current recorded following suprathreshold depolarizations is the Na⁺ current, it

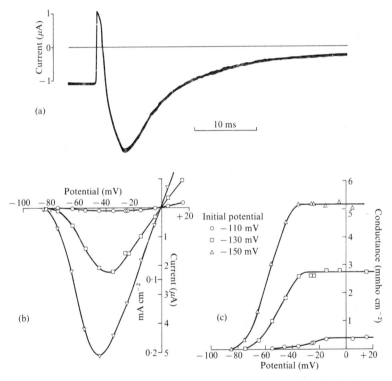

FIG. 4.1. Na⁺ current in cooled Purkinje fibres. (a) Response to depolarization from $-120\ mV$ to $-20\ mV$. An outward capacity current lasting about 2 ms is followed by an inward Na⁺ current. (b) Peak Na⁺ current as a function of membrane potential. The peak inward current is maximal around $-40\ mV$ and is also strongly dependent on the initial potential. (c) Peak Na⁺ conductance as a function of potential. (From Dudel and Rüdel 1970).

is not likely that any of the techniques used so far have succeeded in recording this current accurately in Purkinje fibres or in ventricular muscle (see Beeler and Reuter 1970a; Johnson and Lieberman 1971; New and Trautwein 1972a). The difficulties in doing so arise partly from its rapid speed of onset and partly from its magnitude. The problems arising from the magnitude of the conductance will be discussed at the end of this chapter. The rapid speed of onset raises the problem already mentioned: that the onset of i_{Na^+} overlaps with the decay of i_c.

This problem was partly overcome by Dudel and Rüdel (1970), who studied the Na^+ current at low temperatures where its time-course is greatly slowed. They also avoided some of the problems arising from the magnitude of the current by analysing fibres in which the current was small enough to allow a stable voltage clamp to be achieved.

Fig. 4.1 shows an example of the current records obtained together with current–voltage diagrams showing the peak Na^+ current as a function of membrane potential. As in nerve, the current increases towards a peak inward value as the Na^+ conductance activates. The current then falls as the reversal potential E_{Na^+} is approached. In this case E_{Na^+} lies at $0\,mV$, whereas E_{Na^+} normally lies at about $+40\,mV$. The explanation is that, in the cold, with the ion pumps inactivated, the ion-concentration gradients diminish and so do the reversal potentials. The bottom diagram shows the peak Na^+ conductance as a function of membrane potential calculated using the relation

$$g_{Na^+} = i_{Na^+}/(E_m - E_{Na^+}). \tag{4.1}$$

As in squid nerve, g_{Na^+} increases following a sigmoid curve until a peak value is reached.

The rate constants of activation m and inactivation h were also found to be similar to those in squid, although the inactivation process was not found to follow a simple exponential decay. Dudel and Rüdel were able to fit their results with the Hodgkin–Huxley equation already discussed in Chapter 2,

$$i_{Na^+} = m^3 h \bar{g}_{Na^+} (E_m - E_{Na^+}). \tag{2.9}$$

Fig. 4.2 shows the fit of the equation to the experimental data. This figure may be compared to the squid Na^+ conductance results shown in Fig. 2.4 (p. 25). The resemblance is striking. The empirical functions used by Dudel and Rüdel for the α and β rate coefficients were similar but not identical to those used by Hodgkin and Huxley. The major difference lies in an unusual dependence of h on membrane potential. In the cold,

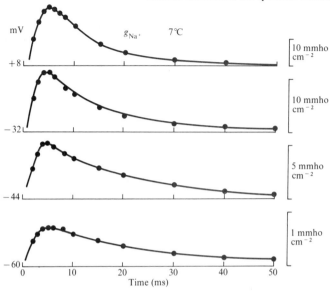

FIG. 4.2. Use of Hodgkin–Huxley equations to reproduce Na^+ conductance changes in Purkinje fibres. The points show experimental measurements. The curves are solutions to the Hodgkin–Huxley equations with appropriately chosen rate coefficients. Note changes in conductance scale (*right*) as the depolarization (*left*) is increased. Compare with Fig. 2.4 (p. 25) (Dudel and Rüdel 1970).

the inactivation curve for Na^+ is shifted to more negative potentials. The reason for this effect is unknown.

Na^+ inactivation and recovery

Apart from the displacement of the inactivation curve at low temperature, the results of Dudel and Rüdel suggest that the inactivation process may be more complex than in normal squid nerve in showing more than one time-constant of decay. The results on other cardiac preparations have proved even more strikingly different. In nerve the recovery from inactivation occurs at a speed not dissimilar to that of the inactivation process. This is expected if the inactivation and recovery processes are the forward and back reactions of a single mechanism (although some voltage-dependence of the reaction rate is expected, it is not usually as large as two orders of magnitude). Thus, in squid, the recovery occurs within a few msecs so that the nerve rapidly becomes re-excitable, i.e. the refractory period is short.

Sodium current and the spread of excitation

By contrast, in atrial muscle Haas, Kern, Einwächter, and Tarr (1971) found that the recovery process may take as long as 400 ms, compared to a few milliseconds for inactivation. Similar results have been obtained in ventricular muscle by Gettes and Reuter (1974). This observation explains the long refractory period in this tissue and may be responsible for the long refractory periods in some other cardiac cells, such as the AV node (Hoffman and Cranefield 1960; Meredith, Mendez, Mueller, and Moe 1968).

From a clinical point of view these observations must be the most interesting made on the Na^+ conductance, since the refractory period may be of importance in some arrhythmias. Thus, the ability of a wave of excitation to return to its origin at a time when the cells are re-excitable may lead to a form of fibrillation. The long refractory period of some regions of the heart may prevent this and anti-arrythmic drugs that prolong the recovery period (see Vaughan-Williams 1971) may owe some of their therapeutic effect to this action.

The magnitude of the Na^+ current

There are two major difficulties concerned with the magnitude of the Na^+ conductance. The first is that it is generally too large to allow controlled voltage-clamp experiments. The second is that the largest Na^+ currents recorded experimentally are too small to account for the speed of depolarization and propagation. As we shall see, these two problems may be connected.

An example of the difficulties involved in maintaining spatial uniformity and control may be given by considering the $1-2$ mm length of Purkinje fibre usually used in voltage-clamp experiments on this preparation (see Chapter 3, p. 40). We will suppose (as shown by Weidmann (1951)) that under normal circumstances the peak Na^+ conductance is at least 100 times as large as the resting membrane conductance. Since the space-constant is proportional to $\sqrt{r_m}$, or $\sqrt{(1/g_m)}$, the 'space-constant' during the conductance increase will be reduced by at least $\sqrt{100}$ i.e. tenfold. Thus a fibre which is 0.25λ long at rest may become 2.5λ long during activity. The non-uniformities produced may then be extremely large.

Strictly speaking, the spatial non-uniformity may not be estimated using simple calculations based on an equation like eqn (3.2) since this equation is obtained by assuming the membrane is represented by a constant resistance. The membrane is then said to be linear since the current—voltage relation is linear. During voltage-dependent conductance changes the membrane behaves in a very non-linear fashion. Nevertheless, the notional decrease in 'space-constant' calculated here gives some idea of the magnitude of the problem.

More realistic calculations may be done using non-linear cable equations in which the membrane current is represented by functions that reproduce the current–voltage relations during excitation (see Jack, Noble and Tsien (1975), Chapter 12). An example of one of these functions is shown in Fig. 4.3(b). The interrupted curve is the assumed form of the ionic current–voltage relation. The continuous curves show the relation between applied current and recorded voltage at the injection point for cables of various lengths D. The curve for $D = 0.5$ (i.e. a fibre half a space-constant long) is not dissimilar to the interrupted curve in shape. As the fibre length is increased, the peak inward current point moves to the left and the curve becomes steeper in the region of threshold. Thus, at $D = 1.5$ the curve is almost vertical near threshold (about 25 mV depolarization). The model used here displays a roughly tenfold increase in conductance (i.e. the conductance at the peak inward current point in the interrupted curve is about 10 times the conductance near the resting potential). Since the actual conductance increase is at least 100-fold, the distance values should be reduced by a factor of about $\sqrt{10}$, i.e. about 3. Serious distortion of the current–voltage relation in real situations might therefore be expected for fibre lengths of about 0.4 space-constants, i.e. for fibre lengths similar to those used experimentally.

Fig. 4.3(a) shows distortion of this type in the Na^+ current–voltage relations obtained experimentally from ventricular muscle. The current–voltage relation shows an almost vertical region near threshold so that the threshold and peak current points are separated by only a few millivolts, compared to a separation of around 40–50 mV in squid nerve fibres. Problems in interpreting the Na^+ current–voltage relations are discussed in more detail by Beeler and Reuter (1970a) and Johnson and Lieberman 1971).

Curiously enough, these distortions are not particularly evident in the Na^+ current–voltage relations for Purkinje fibres shown in Fig. 4.1. They are not completely absent, however. When the Na^+ conductance is partially inactivated (as in the case of the curves drawn through the square and circular points), the voltage at which the peak conductance is reached does shift in a positive direction. Thus, the peak conductance when the Na^+ current is fully available (square symbols) occurs at -40 mV. When the conductance is greatly reduced (circular symbols), the peak conductance occurs at about -15 mV. Nevertheless, this effect is relatively

Sodium current and the spread of excitation

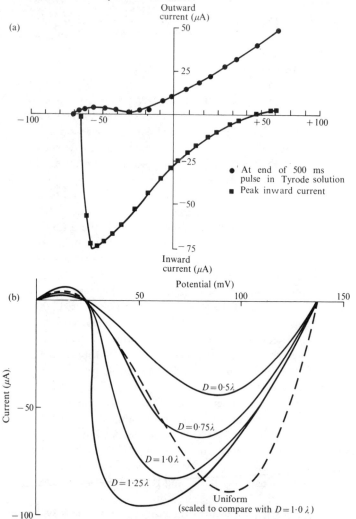

FIG. 4.3. Illustration of Na$^+$-current–voltage relations and difficulties in their interpretation. (a) Current–voltage relations in dog ventricle in normal Tyrode solution. Na$^+$ threshold is at -65 mV. The current then appears to activate fully within only 5 mV (peak inward current is at -60 mV). This compares to an activation range of 60 mV in squid nerve (from Beeler and Reuter 1970*a*). (b) Influence of cable properties on current–voltage relation. The results were calculated assuming a membrane current–voltage relation given by the interrupted line. The continuous curves show relations computed for fibres of various lengths D as shown. As the fibre length is increased, the inward current apparently activates over a narrower range of voltages and the shape of the relation approaches that observed experimentally (from Jack, Noble, and Tsien 1975).

minor compared to that shown by the sharp threshold in the ventricular fibre curve in Fig. 4.3(a).

This suggests that the sodium currents measured in Dudel and Rüdel's experiment may be considerably smaller than those expected from Weidmann's estimate of the conductance increase during the action potential.

There are two reasons for thinking that this is the case. First, the fibres used for analysis were selected as those which allowed stable voltage–clamp experiments to be performed. Fibres in which the Na^+ currents were too large were not used (see Dudel and Rüdel (1970), p. 139). Secondly, the maximum Na^+ currents recorded are too small to account for the maximum depolarization rate in Purkinje fibres if the Na^+ conductance is assumed to be uniformly distributed in the fibre. The amount required to depolarize at the maximum rate of about 800 V s^{-1} may be calculated as shown in Chapter 2, eqn (2.15),

$$1 \times 10^{-6} \, F \, cm^{-2} \times 800 \, V \, s^{-1} = 800 \, \mu A = 0 \cdot 8 \, mA \, cm^{-2}.$$

By contrast, the peak Na^+ current shown in Fig. 4.1 is only 0·2 mA cm^{-2}. (Note that these figures are corrected to give densities of current per unit membrane area using Mobley and Page's estimates of a factor of 10 between total membrane area and that of the fibre surface – see p. 50 above.) This would give a depolarization rate of only about 200 V s^{-1}. This is similar to that obtained using the 1962 model and, as Dudel and Rüdel note, their observed maximum conductance of 50 mS cm^{-2} (1 S = 1 mho) of fibre surface is the same as that used in that model (see Fig. 2.6, p. 29). For this conductance to produce the depolarization and propagation rates observed one must suppose that it discharges only about a quarter of the total capacitance (Noble 1962b).

This suggests a possible solution: that most of the Na^+ conductance is located in the membranes near the surface of a fibre. From a functional point of view this would be the most efficient way of distributing the Na^+ conductance since it is the surface (or near-surface) capacitance C_s that determines the conduction velocity. The rate of discharge of cell membranes deep in the fibre is relatively unimportant. However, we know of no physiological or developmental reasons why the Na^+ conductance should be weak in the membranes of deep cells that are packed close together. Moreover, it may be very difficult to subject the idea to experimental test. In an analogous situation in skeletal muscle, Adrian and Peachey (1973) have shown that the voltage-clamp Na^+ currents may be very insensitive to the amount of Na^+ conductance located in the deep membranes formed by the transverse tubular network.

5 Calcium current and the initiation of contraction

One of the most exciting results of the application of voltage-clamp techniques to cardiac muscle is the finding that there is a smaller and slower inward current carried, at least partly, by calcium ions. The possible involvement of Ca^{2+} current was shown before the use of the voltage-clamp technique (see Niedergerke 1963; Orkand and Niedergerke 1966a). Using the voltage-clamp technique, Reuter (1967) showed that a net inward current could flow across the Purkinje fibre membrane in a Na^+-free solution containing calcium ions. This current has since been investigated by Vitek and Trautwein (1971). The most detailed studies have been done on ventricular (Mascher and Peper 1969; Beeler and Reuter 1970b; New and Trautwein 1972a,b) and atrial fibres (Rougier, Vassort, Garnier, Gargouil, and Coraboeuf 1969). An excellent review of Ca^{2+} currents in excitable membranes has been written by Reuter (1973).

Separation of Na^+ and Ca^{2+} currents

The Ca^{2+} current may be distinguished from the initial Na^+ current in several ways since the conductance mechanisms involved respond differently to blocking drugs and they have a strikingly different dependence on potential and time. Thus the threshold for activating the Ca^{2+} conductance is usually about -30 mV compared to -60 mV for the Na^+ conductance. By holding the membrane potential at -40 mV it is possible to completely inactivate the Na^+ current so that the Ca^{2+} current may then be studied alone. Fig. 5.1 shows current records obtained by Beeler and Reuter (1970b) in an experiment of this kind. The left-hand record shows current recorded in response to a depolarization from -40 mV to -25 mV in the presence of $1\cdot8$ mM Ca^{2+}, the centre record shows the current in Ca^{2+}-free solution, while the right-hand record shows the current obtained after return to $1\cdot8$ mM Ca^{2+} solution. It is evident that depolarization produces an inward current that requires about 200 ms to inactivate (compared to a few milliseconds for Na^+ inactivation — see previous chapter) and that this current is absent in the Ca^{2+}-free solution.

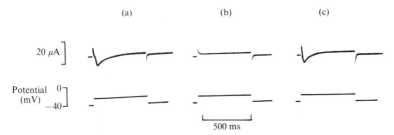

FIG. 5.1. Evidence for Ca^{2+} current in dog ventricle. (a) Response of membrane current (top) to depolarization from $-40\,mV$ to $-25\,mV$ in Tyrode solution containing $1\cdot8\,mM\ Ca^{2+}$. Note presence of transient inward current. (b) Response in $0\,mM\ Ca^{2+}$. Note absence of inward current. (c) Recovery of inward current after readmitting calcium ions to the bathing solution. (Beeler and Reuter 1970b.)

Another way of demonstrating the presence of a second inward current is to measure the current–voltage relations in a Na^+-free solution. Fig. 5.2 shows the current–voltage relations obtained in dog ventricle for the second inward current and the steady outward current. The presence of a net inward current at some potentials in the absence of sodium ions reinforces the conclusion that the second inward current

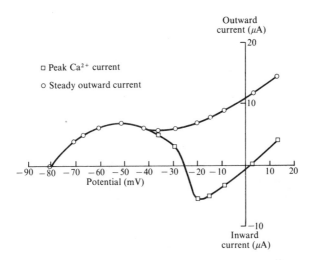

FIG. 5.2. Current–voltage relations showing peak Ca^{2+} current and steady outward current in dog ventricle. Note that threshold (-40 to $-30\,mV$) for activation of Ca^{2+} current is significantly different from that for activation of Na^+ current ($-65\,mV$; see Fig. 4.3, p. 56).

59

Calcium current and the initiation of contraction

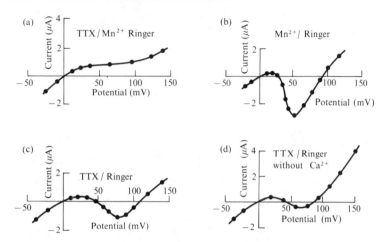

FIG. 5.3. Current–voltage relations from frog atrium showing different sensitivity of Na⁺ and Ca²⁺ currents to tetrodotoxin (TTX) and Mn²⁺. (a) In presence of both blockers, current–voltage diagram shows no net inward current positive to the resting potential.(b) In presence of Mn²⁺, Na⁺ current with threshold 25 mV from resting potential is obtained. (c) In tetrodotoxin Ringer, Ca²⁺ current is recorded with threshold 50 mV from resting potential. (d) In tetrodotoxin Ringer free of calcium ions, some inward current is observed. The 'Ca⁺' channels must therefore also conduct some sodium ions. (Rougier *et al.* 1969.)

is carried by calcium ions. Moreover, a comparison with Fig. 4.3(a) (p. 56) makes it clear that the second inward current is activated at a less negative threshold.

Finally, the Ca²⁺ current and the Na⁺ current may also be distinguished by their differing sensitivities to blocking agents. As in nerve fibres, the initial Na⁺ conductance is blocked by tetrodotoxin. The second inward current is insensitive to tetrodotoxin but is blocked by manganese ions, to which the initial Na⁺ current is insensitive.

Figs 5.3 and 5.4 show current–voltage diagrams and inward current inactivation curves obtained in frog atrium by Rougier, Vassort, Garnier, Gargouil, and Coraboeuf (1969). They found that in the presence of both tetrodotoxin and manganese ions no inward currents are recorded. In the presence of manganese ions, the current–voltage relation shows an inward current with a threshold at about −60 mV (assuming a resting potential equal to −80 mV; see Fig. 3.3, p. 44). Consistent with the view that this is the initial Na⁺ current, the inactivation curve (Fig. 5.4) shows only a fast time-constant of 0·8 ms. In the presence of tetrodotoxin, the inward current is smaller and the threshold now lies at −30 mV.

60

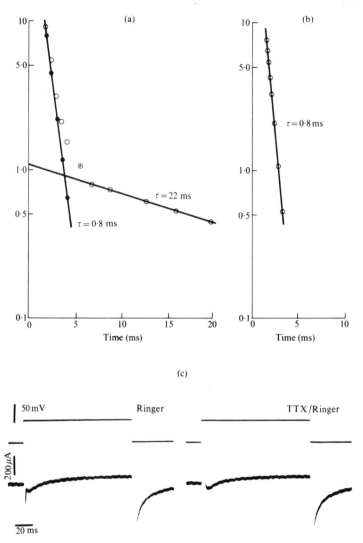

FIG. 5.4. Time-course of inactivation of inward currents in frog atrium. (a) In-activation of current in normal Ringer (○). The current is plotted on a logarithmic scale so that an exponential decay is a straight line. Note the presence of two exponential components. The slow component inactivates with a time-constant τ of 22 ms. Subtraction of this current from the total current gives a component (●) that decays with a time constant of 0·8 ms. (b) In presence of manganese ions, the slow component is absent and only the fast component is found. (Rougier *et al.* 1969.)

Calcium current and the initiation of contraction

The inactivation time-constant is then 22 ms. In the absence of tetrodotoxin and of manganese ions the inactivation process shows two time-constants, 0·8 ms and 22 ms. Finally, we may note that in atrial fibres (though not apparently in ventricular fibres) some inward current flows in the absence of calcium ions even when the initial inward current is blocked by tetrodotoxin. The second inward channel in atrial membrane is not therefore completely specific for calcium ions but may also conduct some sodium ions.

Rougier and Vassort (1971) have shown that the current flow through the second inward channel is determined by the ratio $[Ca^{2+}]/[Na^{+}]^{2}$, which suggests that the sodium and calcium ions compete for the conductance mechanism which can carry two sodium ions in place of one calcium ion (see p. 129). This property resembles the stoichiometry found for the competition between calcium and sodium ions in determining the contraction strength (Lüttgau and Niedergerke 1958; Niedergerke 1963; Orkand and Niedergerke 1966a,b). As we shall see below (p. 64), there is strong evidence to show that the second inward current is involved in triggering contraction so that this resemblance is not surprising.

Role of Ca^{2+} current in maintaining plateau

These results suggest that the role in maintaining the plateau assigned to the residual Na^{+} conductance in the 1962 model (Fig. 2.6, p. 29) is in fact at least partly played by the Ca^{2+} conductance. This changes the model in an important respect since the Ca^{2+} conductance is inactivated much more slowly than the Na^{+} conductance, and this inactivation time-course may contribute to determining the duration of the action potential.

This point may be illustrated by studying the voltage dependence of the rate of inactivation of the Ca^{2+} current. Fig. 5.5 shows the voltage dependence of the inactivation rate in dog ventricular fibres. The rate is fast at very negative potentials but, in the region of the plateau (positive to 0 mV), the inactivation rate is low. The time-constant is about 500 ms in this case (note that this is considerably longer than in frog atrium — Fig. 5.4). This time-constant is comparable with the duration of the ventricular action potential. Hence, there can be little doubt that in ventricular fibres inactivation of the Ca^{2+} current occurs throughout the duration of the plateau. This process therefore plays a kinetic role similar to that of the activation of $g_{K^{+}_2}$ in the 1962 model (Fig. 2.6, p. 29). I shall discuss the kinetic processes of other conductances mechanisms involved in the repolarization process in the next chapter.

It is difficult to overemphasize the importance of the discovery of

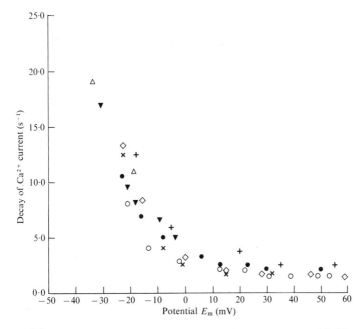

FIG. 5.5. Rate of decay of $i_{Ca^{2+}}$ in ventricular muscle at various potentials. The different symbols refer to different experiments. Note that the decay rate is lowest (i.e. the time-constant is longest) at positive potentials. The Ca^{2+} current therefore decays slowly during the plateau of the ventricular action potential. (Beeler and Reuter 1970b.)

a second inward current mechanism involved in the cardiac action potential. The presence of this component modifies the model described in Fig. 2.6 (p. 29) in several important ways.

The most important modification is that the maintenance of the plateau is relatively independent of the generation of a high conduction velocity. As shown in the previous chapter, the latter is achieved by the very large initial Na^+ conductance. In the 1962 model any change in the magnitude of this conductance would automatically involve a dramatic change in the magnitude and duration of the plateau in addition to changing the conduction velocity. The presence of a second inward component allows a plateau to develop even under conditions in which the rapid initial depolarization is largely absent. In fact, experiments on the action potential have revealed conditions in which either the plateau phase or the initial rapid depolarization can occur independently (Paes de Carvalho, Hoffman, and Paula de Carvalho 1969).

Calcium current and the initiation of contraction

Carmeliet and Vereecke (1969) have described experiments that illustrate the importance of this independence in understanding the action of adrenaline on the action-potential plateau. Adrenaline increases the magnitude of the Ca^{2+} current (see p. 67 below). Thus, in the presence of adrenaline, the plateau is enhanced and it is then possible to obtain an action potential without activating the initial Na^+ conductance. This effect is shown in Fig. 5.6. When the Na^+ current is blocked with

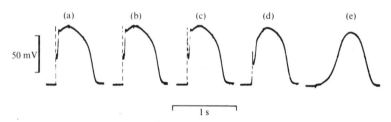

FIG. 5.6. Action potential recorded in calf Purkinje fibres in presence of adrenaline ($5 \cdot 5 \times 10^{-6}$ M). The Na^+ current was progressively blocked with increasing doses of tetrodotoxin: (a) control; (b) 3×10^{-8} M; (c) 3×10^{-7} M; (d) and (e) 3×10^{-6} M. Note complete absence of initial spike in (e). (Carmeliet and Vereecke 1969).

the tetrodotoxin, the depolarization rate is greatly reduced and the 'spike' of the action potential disappears, but the plateau phase remains,

Another consequence of the discovery of a second inward current is that it dispenses with the need to modify the Hodgkin—Huxley Na^+ current equations in the way required in the 1962 model. In this model, the activation m of the Na^+ current was assumed to be less voltage-sensitive than in squid nerve (see Noble (1962a), Fig. 4) in order to satisfy the rather stringent conditions imposed by requiring the Na^+ conductance both to maintain the plateau of the action potential and to provide sufficient inward current at very negative potentials for pacemaker activity to occur (see Chapter 7). Although we cannot be sure that Dudel and Rüdel's Na^+ current records are free from distortion (see Chapter 4), their results do suggest that the activation variable m is as sensitive to potential as it is in nerve. In more recent work on action potential models, the equations for the Na^+ current resemble those of Hodgkin and Huxley more closely (McAllister, Noble, and Tsien 1975).

The initiation of contraction

Ever since Sidney Ringer (1883) observed that extracellular calcium ions are required for contraction to occur in cardiac muscle, it has been realized that Ca^{2+} is important in the initiation of contraction. The observation that the influx of Ca^{2+} increases during activity (Winegrad and Shanes 1962; Niedergerke 1963) suggested that extracellular Ca^{2+} controls contraction by determining the intracellular concentration so that the inward flow of a Ca^{2+} current would be an important link between electrical and mechanical excitation. The use of the voltage-clamp technique has amply confirmed this view.

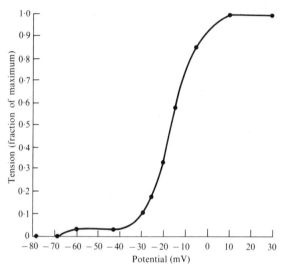

FIG. 5.7. Relation between strength of contraction and membrane potential in ventricular muscle under voltage-clamp conditions (Beeler and Reuter 1970c).

Fig. 5.7 shows the relation between peak tension developed and the membrane potential in a voltage-clamped ventricular muscle (Beeler and Reuter 1970c). A small amount of tension appears at about -60 mV which is the threshold for activating the initial Na^+ current (see Fig. 4.3(a), p. 56) in this preparation. The membrane must then be depolarized by another 30 mV to the threshold for the Ca^{2+} current (see Fig. 5.2) before the tension increases along a sigmoid curve reaching its maximum at about 0 mV. Clearly, the greater part of the contraction is related to the activation of Ca^{2+} inflow. Since the membrane potential is not very effectively controlled during the Na^+ current flow (see Chapter 4, p. 57) it is likely that the small amount of tension appearing at the Na^+ threshold is attributable to Ca^{2+} current flowing in regions that escape the voltage clamp.

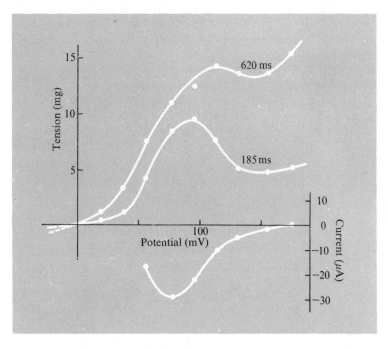

FIG. 5.8. Correlation between Ca^{2+} current and strength of contraction in frog atrial muscle. The contraction rises to a peak as the Ca^{2+} current increases and partially declines when the current decreases as the reversal potential (at a depolarization of 175 mV) is approached. Not all the tension is well correlated with Ca^{2+} current. A maintained component is present and is even more evident at 620 ms than at 185 ms. (Vassort 1973.)

The correlation between Ca^{2+} current and tension is very strikingly illustrated in Fig. 5.8, which shows the results of an experiment on frog atrium in which the peak Ca^{2+} current and the tension are plotted against potential. The tension increases rapidly when the Ca^{2+} current first becomes appreciable at 50 mV depolarization. Assuming a resting potential of −80 mV (see Fig. 3.3, p. 44) this corresponds to a depolarization to −30 mV. The peak tension occurs at a potential similar to that for the peak current and, as the membrane is further depolarized towards the Ca^{2+} equilibrium potential, both the Ca^{2+} current and the tension decline. However, the tension does not decline towards zero as one would expect if Ca^{2+} current entry were the sole factor involved. There is clearly a component of tension that is independent of the Ca^{2+} current. This component becomes even more evident when longer pulses (620 ms) are used. The mechanism of this maintained tension is still controversial (see Morad and Goldman 1973), and I shall restrict this account to the initial tension that is closely related to Ca^{2+} inflow.

Since calcium ions are involved in activating the contractile proteins in muscle (Ebashi and Endo 1968), a very simple hypothesis that is suggested by these observations is that it is the calcium ions that enter the muscle cells during each action potential that activate the contractile machinery.

Unfortunately, this simple hypothesis does not fit some important facts. First, the tension developed is not simply related to the amount of Ca^{2+} entering during *one* action potential. When a series of action potentials occur, it is well known that the peak tension is developed only after several action potentials. This phenomenon is the 'staircase' effect (Niedergerke 1963; Orkand 1968), and it suggests that the Ca^{2+} entering during preceding action potentials is also important in determining the strength of contraction, particularly since it is found that, during the development of the staircase effect, the Ca^{2+} current inflow does not increase. This observation creates a serious difficulty for the theory that the Ca^{2+} current activates contraction directly. A further difficulty is created by the fact that the total amount of Ca^{2+} entering during each action potential is too small to account for the increase in intracellular Ca^{2+} concentration required to produce contraction. It seems more likely, therefore, that the entry of Ca^{2+} during electrical activity is responsible for releasing much larger intracellular stores of Ca^{2+} in the sarcoplasmic reticulum or other intracellular compartments (Bassingthwaite and Reuter 1972; Morad and Goldman 1973).

The action of adrenaline on Ca^{2+} current and contraction

It is well known that one of the major actions of adrenaline on the heart is to increase the force of contraction. This is known as its inotropic action. Since adrenaline has also been found to increase the Ca^{2+} current inflow (Reuter 1967; Rougier *et al.* 1969) it seems likely that part at least of the inotropic action of adrenaline is related to its action on the Ca^{2+} current inflow.

Fig. 5.9 shows an experiment to illustrate this possibility. The experimental setup is similar to that used for Fig. 5.8 and, as in that figure, the tension correlates well with the Ca^{2+} current inflow. When adrenaline is applied, both the Ca^{2+} current and the tension are greatly increased.

In addition to its inotropic action, adrenaline also has a chronotropic action in increasing the frequency of pacemaker activity. The mechanisms

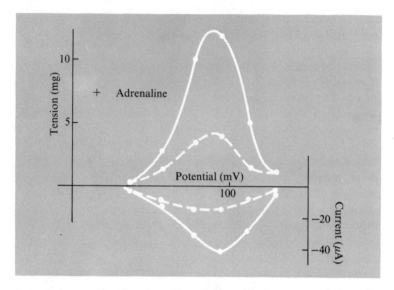

FIG. 5.9. Influence of adrenaline (5 × 10^{-6} M) on strength of contraction and on Ca^{2+} current flow. Both are increased by similar relative amounts. (Vassort 1973.)

of this action will be discussed in Chapter 8 after the mechanisms of pacemaker activity have been described.

6   The repolarization process

The most striking feature of cardiac action potentials when compared with those of other excitable cells, such as nerve and skeletal muscle, is that the repolarization process is extremely slow. In Purkinje fibres the maximum rate of voltage change during the final phase of repolarization is less than 0·5 V s^{-1} (see Fig. 6.1), which is less than 0·1 per cent of the maximum rate of depolarization (800 V s^{-1}). The maximum net current flowing during repolarization is therefore extremely small. In Chapter 1 I discussed the functional significance of this slow rate of repolarization in

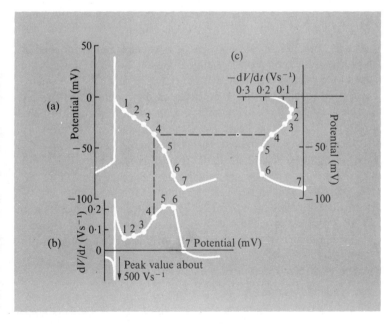

FIG. 6.1. Ionic current-flows during repolarization estimated by measuring the rate of change of potential. At each point the value of dV/dt ($= i_i/C_m$ where C_m is the capacitance of the membrane) is plotted against time (below) and against membrane potential (right). The interrupted lines show an example of the corresponding points (in this case, point 4). During depolarization i_i is very negative (peak value of dV/dt is about 500 V s^{-1}). During repolarization the net ionic current is very much smaller (redrawn from Noble and Tsien (1972)).

The repolarization process

allowing the action potential duration to be large enough to influence the magnitude and duration of contraction. In addition, it ensures a long refractory period (though this function is also served by the slow recovery rate of the Na^+ conductance — see p. 54). Finally, the repolarization rate and its propagation through the heart are important in determining the T wave of the electrocardiogram (see p. 10). As I shall show in Chapter 9 the repolarization rate is very sensitive to factors of clinical importance, such as the plasma K^+ concentration. In view of its importance, it is worth discussing the mechanism of repolarization in some detail, although to do so I shall not be able to adopt the style of previous chapters in leaving the more physical aspects of the subject to the end of the chapter. However, we may greatly simplify the theory by using net current–voltage diagrams and by making use of the fact that the net current and the repolarization rate are closely related by eqn (2.18),

$$-c\frac{dV}{dt} = I_i. \tag{2.18}$$

Strictly speaking, this proportionality between I_i and dV/dt applies only where there is no propagation (see Chapter 2, p. 37). However, the shape of the repolarization phase is not critically dependent on whether propagation occurs. The action potentials in short segments of Purkinje fibre are similar to those in long fibres, apart from the variability that is probably attributable to the damage done in cutting short segments.

It should also be remembered that the shape of the repolarization phase varies considerably in different parts of the heart (see Fig. 1.3, p. 7) and these variations must reflect differences of a quantitative, or even qualitative, kind in the ionic current mechanisms involved. I shall discuss the Purkinje fibre in some detail to illustrate the principles of the analysis. Possible reasons for the different shapes of action potentials elsewhere in the heart will be dealt with towards the end of the chapter.

Net current flow during repolarization

We may illustrate the use of eqn (2.18) by calculating the net ionic current flow as shown in Fig. 6.1. Fig. 6.1(a) shows the action potential with various points during repolarization labelled 1–7. These points are used to label corresponding points in the three diagrams shown. Fig. 6.1(b) shows $-dV/dt$ plotted as a function of time. During depolarization dV/dt is very large and positive for a very brief period of time. This corresponds to the period of intense inward Na^+ current. Following the peak of the action potential there is a relatively fast phase of repolarization (this is highly characteristic of Purkinje fibres and is not found in other parts of the heart – see Fig. 1.3, p. 7). During this phase a moderately large outward current flows. At the beginning of the plateau (point 1) dV/dt and I_i reach minimal values (in some fibres I_i may even become negative again for a brief period to produce the 'notch' that often occurs at this point – see Fig. 6.10). As the rate of repolarization accelerates, I_i increases again and finally falls to zero when repolarization is complete. If pacemaker activity occurs, the net current becomes inward again.

We may also plot I_i as a function of potential as shown in Fig. 6.1(c). The net current is then found to be minimal around -20 mV, reaches a maximum around -60 mV, and falls to zero as the maximum diastolic potential -90 mV is approached. This diagram is the 'effective' current –voltage relation during repolarization. It is very useful in analysing the mechanism of repolarization since, as I shall show later in this chapter, it may be related to the current–voltage relations measured or derived from voltage-clamp experiments. In the simplest possible model of the repolarization process, the ionic current–voltage relation is the same as that plotted in Fig. 6.1(c) and does not change with time (see Fig. 6.3(b)). In more complex models which include time-dependent current changes (Fig. 6.3(a) and (c)), the current–voltage relations obtained from voltage -clamp experiments differ in shape from Fig. 6.1(c) but it is still possible to relate the voltage-clamp relations to the effective relation. Since the voltage is usually plotted as the abscissa in voltage-clamp experiments, Fig. 6.1(c) will be rotated by $90°$ in subsequent figures.

Net conductance changes

We have seen that the slow rate of repolarization means that the net repolarizing current I_i is very small. But it is important to note that this does not necessarily require that the individual ionic currents (I_{Na^+}, I_{K^+}, etc.) should be very small. Since I_i is the sum of the individual currents,

$$I_i = I_{Na^+} + I_{K^+} + I_{Ca^{2+}} + ..., \qquad (6.1)$$

it is conceivable (although unlikely in view of the waste of energy involved) that the small net value of I_i results from a fine balance between very large, but opposite, values of inward and outward currents. Thus, in place of the model described in Fig. 2.6 (p. 29), we might use one in which g_{Na^+} does not inactivate rapidly, so that g_{Na^+} remains high during the plateau and requires a large increase in g_{K^+} to overcome the resulting inward current. Such a theory would require a high conductance during the plateau, a large exchange of sodium and potassium ions running down their concentration gradients, and a large energy expenditure by the Na^+-K^+ pump (see Chapter 2) to restore the gradients. By contrast, theories that minimize the energy cost of the action potential require low conductances.

An experiment by Weidmann (1951) to distinguish between these possibilities is shown in Fig. 6.2. The top records show a number of superimposed action potentials. During these responses, the membrane was subjected to a repetitive series of small negative current pulses which produce voltage deflections away from the normal time-course of the repolarization phase. The magnitudes of these deflections depend on the membrane conductance. The smaller the membrane conductance, the larger the voltage deflection since a small conductance corresponds to a large resistance to current flow. Since the pulse frequency was not synchronized with the action-potential frequency, the pulses occur at different times during each action potential. When the action potentials are superimposed, the result is a 'band' of voltage deflections whose amplitude increases as the measured conductance decreases. Since fairly small current pulses were used, the conductance measured is that for small current deflections at each point and will approximate the 'slope' conductance dI_i/dV, i.e. the ratio of the small current applied to the voltage deflection produced.

The continuous curve in the lower diagram in Fig. 6.2 shows the values calculated by Weidmann from this experiment. The precise interpretation of the measurements is complex. The problems involved have been described by Noble and Tsien (1972) and the interrupted curve shows a possible time-course for the slope conductance suggested by Noble and Tsien that includes negative values of conductance and which is also consistent with Weidmann's results. Whichever curve is used the main result is quite clear: the slope conductance during the plateau is very small. This allows us to exclude a fairly simple modification of the Hodgkin–Huxley theory described by FitzHugh (1960) and George and Johnson (1961). They showed that a plateau during the repolarization phase could occur simply by reducing the speed and magnitude of the K^+ conductance in Hodgkin and Huxley's theory. This allows the residual Na^+ conductance (see Chapter 2) to maintain depolarization for a considerable period time. However, as shown by FitzHugh's (1960) work, the plateau slope conductance in this model is larger than the resting conductance.

The explanation for the low value of the plateau conductance in cardiac muscle lies in an important property of the K^+ conductance which

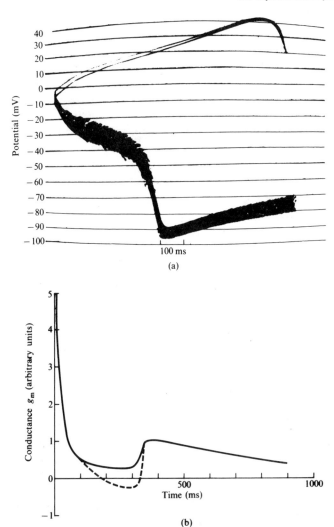

FIG. 6.2. Variation in 'slope' conductance during Purkinje fibre action potential.
(a) Voltage deflections produced by small current pulses applied repetitively during
the action potential. The record shows a number of superimposed traces and,
since the current pulses were not synchronized with the action potentials, the
result is a 'band' of voltage deflections from which estimates of conductance may
be made. (Weidmann 1951.) (b) Continuous curve shows conductance values
obtained by Weidmann (1956). The interrupted curve shows a possible time-course
for conductance that is also consistent with experimental results (Noble and Tsien
1972). Note that, on either interpretation, the slope conductance is very low, and
may be negative, during the plateau. (Noble and Tsien 1972.)

73

The repolarization process

has already been referred to in Chapter 2 (p. 27): when the membrane is depolarized the K^+ conductance initially falls as a result of the inward-rectifying property of the K^+ channels. In consequence, a much smaller inward current is required to maintain the depolarization. The conductances to both outward and inward currents are thus much smaller than would be the case if the K^+ channels did not show inward rectification. It is likely therefore that inward rectification is functionally important in cardiac muscle in minimizing the energy requirements of the action potential

Current—voltage relations during repolarization

The results discussed so far set limits on the magnitude of the currents and conductances during repolarization but they do not allow us to distinguish between several possible interpretations of the effective current—voltage relation plotted in Fig. 6.1(c). In particular, they do not allow us to determine the relative contributions of voltage-dependent and time-dependent changes in the ionic current. In nerve membranes, this distinction would be somewhat artificial since the voltage dependence of the current arises from the voltage-dependence of the opening and closing rates of the ionic gating processes (Chapter 2, p. 22). In cardiac muscle, however, the distinction is important since a considerable fraction of the repolarizing current is carried by channels (e.g. i_{K^+1} — see Chapter 9) that display strong voltage-dependence but no significant time-dependence.

Fig. 6.3 shows that there are large differences between the possible models. Fig. 6.3(a) illustrates the $I_i(V)$ relations that would occur if the current changes were almost entirely time-dependent. This is similar to a model discussed by Johnson and Tille (1961)[†] and Woodbury (1961). Fig. 6.3(b) shows the opposite extreme: the ionic current is purely voltage dependent and the $I_i(V)$ relation does not change with time. This model is not implausible since the shape of the effective current—voltage diagram during repolarization is very similar to that of the time-independent K^+ current i_{K^+1} (see Fig. 9.3, p. 121). Fig. 6.3(c) shows a compromise in which each current—voltage relation is highly non-linear but in which the shape of the relation also changes with time. At early times during the plateau the current—voltage curve is assumed to contain a substantial component of inward Na^+ or Ca^{2+} current so that at some potentials the net ionic current is inward.

[†] Johnson and Tille (1961) actually used linear current—voltage relations but their experimental results do not necessarily show this (see Noble 1962c).

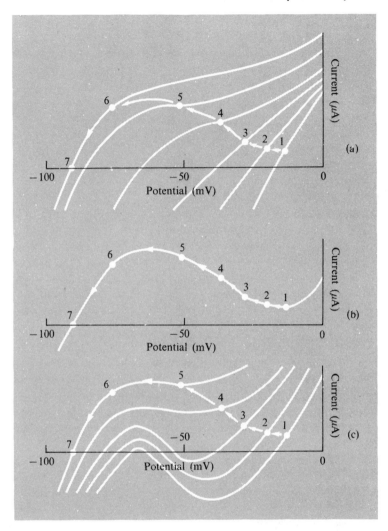

FIG. 6.3. Possible mechanisms of repolarization. (a) Current–voltage relations are assumed to intersect once with the voltage axis and this intersection point moves towards more negative values with time. (b) Current–voltage relation is assumed to be independent of time. The relation then has the same shape as the 'effective' relation during repolarization (see Fig. 6.1(c)). (c) Early current–voltage relations show region of net inward current and intersect the axis at three potentials. The relation loses this inward region as inward current inactivates and outward current increases. (Noble and Tsien 1972.)

The repolarization process

We may note that in each case it is possible to account for the effective current–voltage relation (Fig. 6.1(c)) and for Weidmann's conductance measurements (Fig. 6.2). In cases (a) and (c) the precise course followed by the repolarization process depends on the kinetics assumed for the time-dependent change in the current–voltage relation. An example of case (c) will be described below (Fig. 6.9). In case (b), the course of repolarization is automatically given by the current–voltage relation, as we have already noted.

The conductance changes may be derived from the slopes of the current–voltage diagram at each point during repolarization. In (a), the slope is large (i.e. a large conductance would be measured by small currents) at point 1, reaches a minimum near point 5, and then increases again. This case therefore gives a conductance curve similar to the continuous line in Fig. 6.2(b). In (b), the slope becomes negative between points 2 and 5, to return to positive values at 6 and 7. This behaviour would be similar to the interrupted curve in Fig. 6.2(b). The slopes for case (c) are similar to those of case (a). Thus, although the details vary, the results of each of the models are consistent with those of Weidmann's experiment and some further experimental tests are required to distinguish between them.

All-or-nothing repolarization

Although the mechanisms illustrated in Fig. 6.3 do not differ greatly in their response to small currents, they clearly will differ in their responses to large applied currents since these will deflect the membrane potential into regions where the current–voltage diagrams differ very markedly. This may be illustrated by considering the way in which the responses to brief but large hyperpolarizing currents will differ (Fig. 6.4). We will consider currents of two different strengths (A and B) applied at the point 2 just after the beginning of the plateau. In case (a), both currents will hyperpolarize the membrane into a negative (depolarizing) current region. When the current pulse is terminated the potential will return in a depolarizing direction to the plateau. The pulse will have no significant effect on the subsequent time-course of repolarization. In case (b), exactly the opposite result will be obtained. Both currents hyperpolarize to a region of outward (repolarizing) current so that the repolarization process will simply continue when the pulse is terminated. The duration will be shortened by an amount that depends on the magnitude of the hyperpolarizing current.

In the case of mechanism (c), a more complex result is expected. A small current will deflect the membrane potential to an inward current

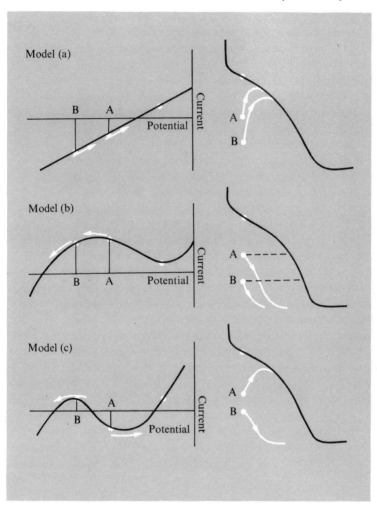

FIG. 6.4. Predicted effects on the models in Fig. 6.3 of brief hyperpolarization. Model (a) generates inward currents in response to all hyperpolarizations beyond the intersection point. Hence, when the pulse is terminated, the membrane depolarizes back to the plateau. In model (b) outward currents are generated so that the membrane hyperpolarizes. In model (c) small hyperpolarizing pulse generates inward current whereas large pulse generates outward current. The middle intersection point forms a threshold beyond which hyperpolarization occurs. (Noble and Tsien 1972.)

region so that depolarization back to the plateau will occur at the end of the pulse. The larger current will deflect the potential *beyond* the region of inward current. Outward (repolarizing) current will flow and the action potential will be shortened. The intersection point at which the current changes direction is a critical voltage that determines the threshold for the all-or-nothing repolarization response.

The crucial question, of course, is what happens when this experiment is performed on cardiac muscle. In the case of ventricular and Purkinje fibres, the result is quite clear: all-or-nothing repolarization does occur (see Fig. 6.10). Mechanism (c) must therefore be operating and over some period of time during the plateau the current–voltage relations must contain a restricted region of inward current.

This may also be demonstrated by using the voltage-clamp technique. Fig. 6.5 (a) and (b) illustrates the result that would be expected when a fibre is clamped at potentials that move stepwise in a depolarizing direction. I have assumed (as shown – Fig. 6.7) that the time-dependent current change that is responsible for shifting the net current in an outward direction is activated at potentials beyond -40 mV. Up to this potential, therefore, the current changes would be expected to follow the ionic current–voltage relation corresponding to the beginning of the plateau ($1 \rightarrow 2 \rightarrow 3$), so that while the potential moves stepwise in a positive direction the current moves in a negative direction. When the threshold for outward current change is reached, the response to each step will be more complex. The initial change may still be inward ($3 \rightarrow 4$) but will be followed by a time-dependent outward change ($4 \rightarrow 5$). Later steps ($5 \rightarrow 6$ $\rightarrow 7$ and $7 \rightarrow 8 \rightarrow 9$) will produce initial and delayed outward changes.

Fig. 6.5(b) shows the result of such an experiment on a Purkinje fibre. The expected results are indeed obtained. It should be noted however that the success of the experiment is partly dependent on the threshold for outward current change being at potentials positive to the negative slope region of the net current–voltage relation. This situation does not always occur and, when the outward current threshold is more negative, net steady-state inward current is more difficult to demonstate.

Role of Ca^{2+} current in repolarization

The results described so far impose two requirements on the ionic current mechanisms involved in repolarization. First, there must exist a net inward current over some potential ranges during the early stages of repolarization. As we have seen in the previous chapter, this current is

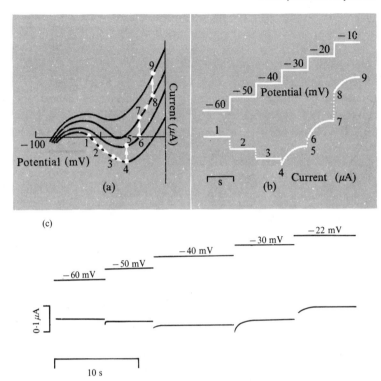

FIG. 6.5. Current changes expected during progressively increasing voltage-clamp steps for model (c). Fig. 6.3. (a) Current–voltage relations during repolarization. The figures 1–9 indicate current changes expected in response to voltage steps assuming that the threshold for activating outward current is between −40 and −30 mV. (b) Corresponding voltage and current changes plotted against time. (c) Experimental record obtained during step depolarizations in a Purkinje fibre. (Noble and Tsien 1972.)

provided largely by the Ca^{2+} current and, to a lesser extent, the residual Na^+ current.

Secondly, beyond a certain potential the current must slowly change in an outward direction. This time-dependent change might result from inward current inactivation or from the activation of outward K^+ current. It seems likely that both processes contribute and that their relative importance varies between different parts of the heart. Thus, in ventricular muscle, the Ca^{2+}.inactivation process is slow ($\tau = 400$ ms, see p. 62), while the activation of outward current is relatively small. In Purkinje fibres, the Ca^{2+} inactivation process is much faster ($\tau = 50$ ms; Vitek and

Trautwein (1971)) and can only be the rate-determining process in action potentials of short duration (e.g. less than 300 ms). In longer action potentials (e.g. Fig. 6.10) the activation of K^+ current is more important. In atrial muscle, the Ca^{2+} inactivation process is even faster (see p. 61). Moreover, although activation of outward K^+ current also occurs, it contributes a relatively small part of the total repolarizing current compared to that provided by the time-independent (background) K^+ current $i_{K^+,1}$ (Hemptinne 1971).

K^+-conductance mechanisms in repolarization

The experiment illustrated in Fig. 6.6 investigates the outward current mechanisms in the Purkinje fibre by carrying the analysis of the experiment shown in Fig. 6.5(b) a stage further. The membrane potential was held at -30 mV, which from Fig. 6.5(b) is about 10 mV beyond the threshold for activating outward current changes. The membrane was then subjected to depolarizing and hyperolarizing current pulses of different magnitudes. Depolarizations (to -20 mV and -10 mV) activate outward currents that increase with the magnitude of the depolarization. Hyperpolarizations to -50 mV and to -70 mV switchoff the current. At -80 mV the current record is nearly flat despite the fact that conductance decay is occurring (a recovery of current similar to that shown on return from -50 mV was observed at the end of the pulse). The reversal potential for the outward current therefore lies at about -80 mV.[†]

This potential differs very significantly from the K^+ equilibrium potential, which lies at about -100 mV (see Chapter 7, p. 94) when $[K^+]_o$ $= 4$ mM. This means that, although potassium ions are largely involved, there must be some contribution from other ions, such as Na^+. To indicate this 'impurity' in the selectivity of the channels, the current was labelled i_x.

It is also clear from Fig. 6.6 that i_x is not controlled by a single time-constant process. The time-course of current on return from -50 mV to -30 mV is noticeably faster than that on return from -10 mV to the same holding potential. When the current changes during the following depolarization to -10 mV are plotted on semi-logarithmic coordinates (Fig. 6.6, bottom) the curves may be fitted by two exponential processes, which means that the current may be represented as the sum of two components,

$$i_x = i_{x,1} + i_{x,2}, \tag{6.2}$$

[†] The fibre used for this analysis showed very little pacemaker current, $i_{K^+,2}$ (see Chapter 7) so that little or no interference by this component occurred.

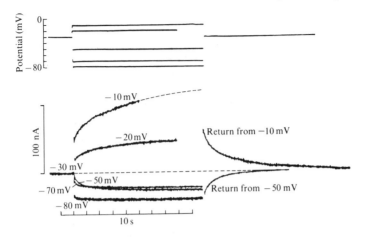

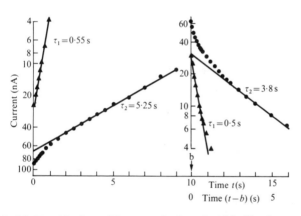

FIG. 6.6. *Top*: Membrane K^+ currents in sheep Purkinje fibre in response to step changes in potential from holding potential of -30 mV. Depolarizations to -20 mV and -10 mV produce slow increases in outward current. Hyperpolarizations decrease the current. Note that the record is nearly flat at -80 mV. *Bottom*: Semi-logarithmic plot of current onset and decay during and following depolarization to -10 mV. Note that record may be analysed into two exponential components. (Noble and Tsien 1969a.)

where $i_{x,1}$ is the fast component ($\tau_{x,1}$ at -30 mV $= 0.5$ s) and $i_{x,2}$ is the slow component ($\tau_{x,2}$ at -30 mV $= 3.8$ s).

In each case, the current changes may be described using equations like (2.5) (see p. 22), where y is replaced by the activation variables x_1 and x_2. The voltage dependence of x_1 and x_2 and of the corresponding

81

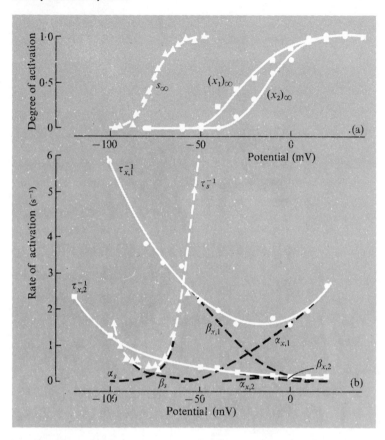

FIG. 6.7. Kinetics of K$^+$ currents in Purkinje fibre (see text). (a) Variation of degrees of activation x_1 and x_2 with potential. (b) Variation of rates of activation or deactivation with potential. The interrupted lines in each case show the kinetics of the pacemaker K$^+$ current $i_{K^+, 2}$ described in the next chapter (p. 93). (From Noble and Tsien 1969b.)

rates of formation ($\alpha_{x,1}, \alpha_{x,2}$) and decay ($\beta_{x,1}, \beta_{x,2}$) of the channels are plotted in Fig. 6.7. As in Hodgkin and Huxley's model of the nerve-impulse currents, these parameters may be used to estimate the contribution of i_x to the total ionic current flow.

Reconstruction of the repolarization process

First, we may calculate the ionic current flow in the absence of i_x by subtracting the steady-state values of $i_{x,1}$ and $i_{x,2}$ from the total steady state current. This procedure should give the current–voltage relation before the activation of i_x, which should resemble the lowest curve in Fig. 6.3(c). This expectation is confirmed in the result shown in Fig. 6.8, from which we can see that the activation of $i_{x,1}$ alone is quite sufficient to abolish the region of net inward (depolarizing) current and so allow repolarization to occur. It is also clear from the time-constants that x_1 is likely to be the important component functionally since its time-constant (0·5 s) is similar to the duration of the action potential. By contrast, the time-constant for x_2 (about 4 s) is much longer than normal action potentials in Purkinje fibres.

Second, we may now use the current–voltage relation $i_0(E_m)$ obtained in Fig. 6.8, together with the measured kinetics of x_1, to estimate how the

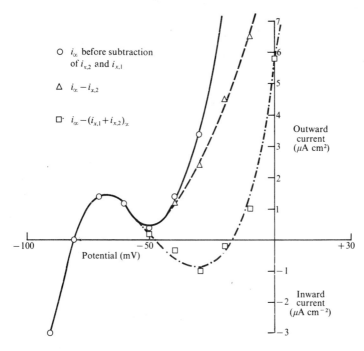

FIG. 6.8. Current–voltage relations before and after subtraction of $i_{x,2}$ and $i_{x,1}$. (Noble and Tsien 1969a.)

total ionic current ($i_0 + i_{x,1}$) will vary during normal activity. Thus, we may start a calculation of the repolarization process using the conditions that $x_1 = 0$ at the beginning of the plateau and $E_m = -9$ mV (which was the observed potential at the beginning of the plateau in the fibre used for analysis). dV/dt may then be calculated as in eqn (2.18), which, for this case, gives

$$dV/dt = (i_0)/c. \qquad (6.3)$$

With time, $i_{x,1}$ will activate, so that subsequent values of dV/dt will be given by

$$dV/dt = (i_0 + i_{x,1})/c. \qquad (6.4)$$

Fig. 6.9 shows the results of such a reconstruction of the repolarization process in which eqn. (6.4) was used to calculate dV/dt at 20 ms intervals. Each value of dV/dt allows us to estimate the change in V over the 20 ms interval which then gives us a new value of V for the next step in the calculation. The top curve (....) shows the reconstructed plateau and repolarization. The bottom curve shows the same results plotted as dV/dt against V to obtain a curve similar to that obtained in Fig. 6.1(c). In addition we have plotted the net current–voltage relations at 100 ms intervals obtained by adding i_0 and $i_{x,1}$ together. These relations clearly resemble the set of relations drawn in Fig. 6.3(c). A region of net inward current persists for about 300 ms. During this time, therefore, the responses to current pulses will resemble those drawn in Fig. 6.4(c). The voltage threshold V_{Th} for all-or-nothing repolarization will be given by the middle intersection points and their values are plotted as the triangles in the upper diagram of Fig. 6.9. The threshold lies at about -60 mV at the beginning of the plateau and approaches -30 mV at 300 ms. These values are similar to those obtained in Vassalle's experimental record (Fig. 6.10).

This reconstruction is clearly highly simplified since all ionic currents apart from $i_{x,1}$ are represented by the single current–voltage relation i_0. This assumes that during processes as slow as repolarization the ionic currents follow steady-state values. This will be valid for the Na^+ current since it activates and inactivates very quickly. However, the Ca^{2+} current inactivates more slowly and in Purkinje fibres its inactivation time-course will be important during the first 100 ms ($\tau_{inact} = 50$ ms; see p. 79). More recently, a complete model of the ionic currents has been constructed (McAllister, Noble and Tsien 1975) which includes the kinetics of $i_{Ca^{+2}}$. The action potential and all-or-nothing repolarization responses given by this model are shown in Fig. 6.10(b), where they may be compared with Vassalle's experimental record (Fig. 6.10(a)).

As in the simpler model, the threshold for all-or-nothing repolarization

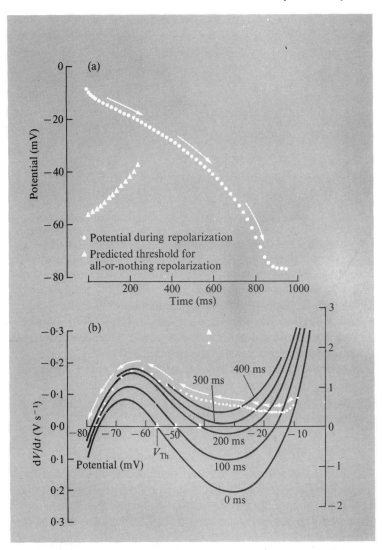

FIG. 6.9. Reconstruction of the repolarization process. (a) Variation of potential during repolarization and of the predicted thesholds for all-or-nothing repolarization. (b) Current−voltage relations during repolarization. The points show the values of V and I_i calculated at 20-ms intervals (same points as in (a)). This resembles the trajectory of repolarization shown in Figs 6.1(c) and 6.3. Curves are current−voltage relations at 100-ms interval. An inward current region persists for about 300 ms. Note resemblance of curves to Fig. 6.3(c). (Noble and Tsien 1969b.)

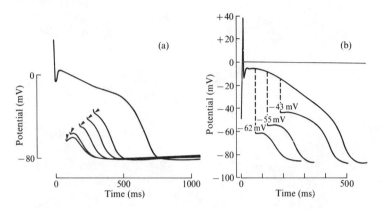

FIG. 6.10. (a) All-or-nothing threshold responses obtained experimentally by Vassalle (1966). (b) Computed responses using model based on voltage-clamp measurements of ionic currents. (McAllister, Noble, and Tsien 1975.)

disappears after 300 ms. After this time, the fibre obeys a set of current —voltage relations similar to those drawn in Fig. 6.3(a), i.e. they are time-dependent but have no net inward current regions in the plateau range of potentials. As I have already explained (Fig. 6.4(a)), all-or-nothing repolarization thresholds do not exist in this case. The responses to hyperpolarizing currents are then graded.

The relative durations of the 'all-or-nothing' and 'graded' phases of the plateau, of course, may vary in different parts of the heart. Short atrial action potentials may have a much shorter 'all-or-nothing' phase than longer Purkinje or ventricular action potentials.

Influence of frequency of beating

One of the ways in which the heart's output may be increased is to increase the frequency at which it beats. It is then important that the relative durations of systole and diastole should be adjusted to ensure that both filling and ejection occur efficiently. Thus an increase in frequency without any change in the duration of systole would lead to a disproportionate decrease in the duration of diastole and, at high frequencies, the ventricles would not be filled before contracting. This problem is avoided by using a property of the excitation-coupling process that I have already referred to (p. 9); the duration of contraction is related to the duration of the action potential. If the action-potential duration decreases at high frequencies so will the duration of systole.

It has long been known that this is the case (for literature on early work see Hoffman and Cranefield (1961)). Thus, if a second action potential is initiated soon after the first, the second is found to be considerably shorter. The relationship between the interval between two action potentials and the duration of the second one is known as the interval—duration relation.

As shown earlier in this chapter, the duration of the action potential depends on the rate of Ca^{2+} current inactivation and of activation of the K^+ current $i_{x,1}$. At the end of the action potential these processes return to their resting state. The Ca^{2+} current becomes reavailable and the K^+ current decays. If an action potential is initiated before these recovery processes are complete, the duration will be shorter than usual since less inward current will be activated and some of the outward current will already be activated.

According to this explanation, the time-scale of the interval—duration relation should be determined by the rate of the recovery processes. In Purkinje fibres the time-constant of the major part of the interval—duration relation is about 200 ms (Fig. 6.11) which is similar to the decay time constant of x_1 at negative potentials. The contribution of the Ca^{2+} recovery process is less certain since there is some disagreement in the literature concerning the time course of recovery. It seems likely, however, that this process is also involved.

Once again it is important to remember the varying contributions of Ca^{2+} inactivation and K^+ activation to the control of action potential duration in different parts of the heart. These differences will be reflected in different relative contributions to the interval—duration relation.

The action of adrenaline on repolarization

As shown in the preceding chapter (p. 67) adrenaline may greatly increase the magnitude of the Ca^{2+} current. By itself this would increase the duration of the action potential since a larger degree of K^+ activation would be required to overcome the depolarizing action of the Ca^{2+} current. Since adrenaline also greatly increases the frequency of beating (see Chapter 8) the result would be a longer systole and a greatly reduced diastole.

This situation is avoided by an additional action of adrenaline on the K^+ current $i_{x,1}$. Tsien, Giles, and Greengard (1972) have shown that in Purkinje fibres $i_{x,1}$ is increased and its activation threshold is shifted to more negative potentials. As a result, the activation of $i_{x,1}$ is greatly

The repolarization process

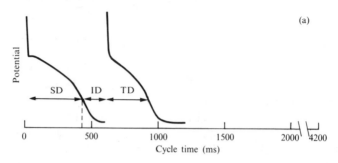

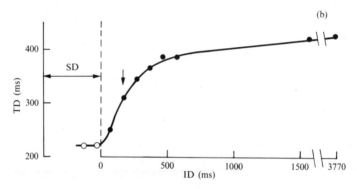

FIG. 6.11. Dependence of action-potential duration on the interval between successive action potentials. (a) Example of experimental record. The first action potential was initiated after at least 10 s rest. Its duration (SD) was about 450 ms. The second action potential was initiated after an interval (ID) and its duration (TD) is plotted in (b) against the interval duration. Note that recovery of action potential duration is initially quite rapid and the 'time-constant' (indicated by arrow) is similar to the decay time-constant of x_1. (Hauswirth, Noble, and Tsien 1972a.)

increased during repolarization. This effect is sufficiently large to ensure that repolarization occurs *more* quickly despite the increased Ca^{2+} current flow. This achieves the functionally desirable result that the duration of the action potential decreases when the frequency is increased by adrenaline.

It is also found that adrenaline increases the mechanical relaxation rate, probably by stimulating Ca^{2+} uptake by intracellular stores (see Chapter 2, p. 18). This effect, together with the reduction in action-potential duration, will ensure that the duration of systole is reduced as the frequency increases.

7 Potassium currents and pacemaker activity

The origin of spontaneous rhythmic activity in the heart has always fascinated physiologists, partly because of its intrinsic importance in the functioning of the body but also because there is a very obvious challenge to the investigator in a process that is spontaneously repetitive. The system cannot simply be transforming or amplifying energy applied to it in the form of stimuli; it must be controlling the flow and dissipation of its own energy stores in a cyclic fashion. Such processes have not only interested physiologists. Their fascination has also attracted physicists and mathematicians to speculate on the action of the heart. Thus, one of the first applications of van der Pol's (1926) mathematical theory of the valve oscillator was to cardiac pacemaker activity (van der Pol and van der Mark 1928). This analogy, like many others born of physical models, has its virtues but also has serious limitations when applied to excitable cells (see Jack, Noble, and Tsien (1975), Chapter 11). It has also been clear since Huxley's (1969) work on repetitive activity in nerve fibres that semi-empirical models of the Hodgkin–Huxley kind are inherently capable of explaining rhythmic firing in excitable cells. The modification of this theory that I described in 1962 (Fig. 2.6, p. 29) reproduced cardiac pacemaker potentials similar to those recorded experimentally.

Notwithstanding the success of these models, the subject forms treacherous ground for theoretical speculation. The facts of nature have a habit of littering the scientific scene with shipwrecked theories. This much we are all familiar with and accept as the virtue of the scientific method. Nevertheless, the manner in which the natural world disposesses us of even our most elegant ideas still takes us by surprise. Who would have predicted a few years ago that the K^+ current controlling pacemaker activity in Purkinje fibres has virtually no influence on the action potential itself? Or that the Purkinje fibre is a misleading model of atrial pacemaker activity? Or that adrenaline should control these two pacemaker regions in the heart by quite different ionic mechanisms? In this chapter and in Chapter 8 I shall describe the experimental work that has led to these conclusions.

Potassium currents and pacemaker activity

The pacemaker potential and its sensitivity to temperature

First, however, we must describe the potential changes that generate rhythmic firing. As in previous chapters I shall start by using the Purkinje fibre as an example. The important differences noted above will be analysed later in the chapter.

Fig. 7.1 shows pacemaker activity recorded at various temperatures

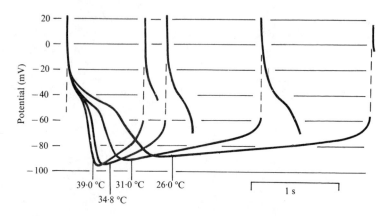

FIG. 7.1. Pacemaker potentials recorded in sheep Purkinje fibre. The figure on each record is the bath temperature. (Weidmann 1956.)

in sheep Purkinje fibres. The potential at which the pacemaker depolarization commences is somewhat temperature dependent and lies between −88 mV and −95 mV. The threshold for the activation of the Na^+ current (indicated roughly by the potential at which the depolarization rate becomes too fast to be recorded by the oscilloscope) lies at −60 mV. I shall therefore refer to the 'pacemaker range' of potentials in Purkinje fibres as lying between −90 mV and −60 mV.

The rate of depolarization during the pacemaker potential is highly temperature-dependent. We usually express the temperature-dependence of biological processes by a parameter known as the Q_{10}, which is the ratio of the rates at two temperatures differing by 10 °C. A 10 °C change in temperature (26–36°C) produces a sixfold change in the rate of depolarization. The process whose rate limits the speed of pacemaker activity must therefore have the relatively high Q_{10} of 6. This property of pacemaker activity in the heart is important in cardiac surgery where low temperatures are used to arrest the heart and so allow operations to be performed on it more easily. In cold-blooded animals, the temperature-dependence of pacemaker activity is also important physiologically. The metabolic demands greatly increase with body temperature, and the heart-rate automatically increases to meet these demands. In mammals, the body temperature is normally controlled within narrow limits, although temperature induced cardiac acceleration occurs in fever when the body temperature rises significantly.

The 'pacemaker range' of potentials in sino-atrial and atrial tissue is significantly different from that in Purkinje fibres. Thus, in frog sinus (see Fig. 1.3(a), p. 7) the range is between -60 mV and -40 mV, which is entirely positive to the range in Purkinje fibres. Pacemaker activity induced in atrial tissue by depolarizing currents also occurs at a more depolarized range of potentials (-65 mV to -45 mV in Fig. 7.8). The significance of this difference between sino-atrial tissue and Purkinje fibres will become apparent later.

What changes in ionic current flow might generate a slow depolarization? An increase in a depolarizing current, such as the Na^+ current, would obviously depolarize the membrane. Likewise, a decrease in a repolarizing (K^+) current would allow a constant (or background) depolarizing current to become dominant. Finally, it is conceivable that the activity of ionic pumps (see Chapter 2) might contribute since (as noted on p. 17), the Na^+-K^+ pump usually carries a net hyperpolarizing current. If the pump displayed maximal activity at the end of the action potential then slowly declined with time, a slow depolarization would result. We may distinguish between these three possibilities by measuring the reversal potential of the current change that generates pacemaker activity. A K^+-current change would show a negative reversal potential a Na^+-current change would have a positive reversal potential, while an electrogenic pump current is unlikely to show a reversal potential. The pump would produce a hyperpolarizing current at all potentials unless a negative potential large enough to counter the energy of the pump were applied. Potentials within the range of physiological experiments do not achieve this situation in the case of the electrogenic pump in nerve membranes (Ritchie 1973). The evidence I shall discuss below shows that the current change controlling the rate of pacemaker activity reverses near the K^+ equilibrium potential (Fig. 7.4). We can be fairly certain therefore that K^+-current changes are involved.

Pacemaker K^+ current in Purkinje fibres

We may measure the current change responsible for the pacemaker potential by clamping the membrane at a potential within the pacemaker range. Thus, if the membrane potential is held constant at −90 mV as soon as this potential is reached at the end of repolarization, the current recorded becomes progressively more inward with time (Vassalle 1966). This net change in current in an inward direction would have depolarized the membrane in the absence of a voltage clamp. By clamping the membrane at a variety of potentials within the pacemaker range it is found that the mechanism responsible for the pacemaker current change is very sensitive to the membrane potential between −90 mV and −60 mV.

Fig. 7.2 shows the results of an experiment of this kind. The membrane

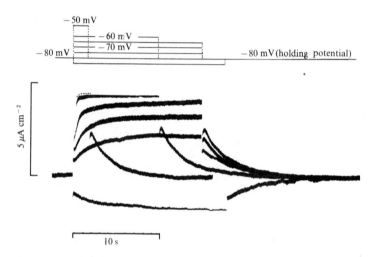

FIG. 7.2. K⁺ currents in a sheep Purkinje fibre in response to step voltage changes in pacemaker range. Outward current is shown as an upward deflection. Six records have been superimposed. (Noble and Tsien 1968.)

potential was initially clamped at −80 mV. A 5 mV depolarization to −75 mV produces an appreciable slow outward current change, and a 5 mV hyperpolarization produces a slow inward current change. Larger depolarizations (10 mV and 15 mV) activate larger outward currents, and the decay tails on return to −80 mV are also larger. This increase in activation occurs over a very narrow range of potentials since the decay tail following 20 mV depolarization (to −60 mV) is no larger than that following 15 mV depolarization. Although not shown in Fig. 7.2, the recovery tails following hyperpolarizations reach a maximum following hyperpolarizations to −90 mV. The activation range of the gating mechanism (−90 mV to −60 mV) is thus virtually the same as the pacemaker

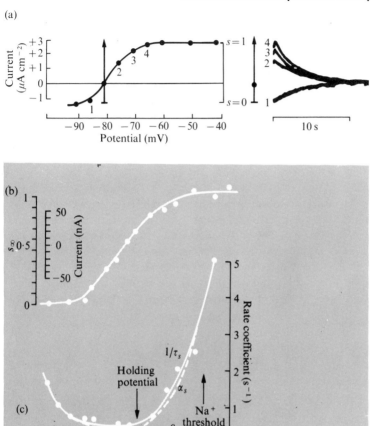

FIG. 7.3. Kinetics of potassium current $i_{K^+, 2}$ in sheep Purkinje fibres. (a) Illustration of the way in which the steady-state activation curve s_∞ is obtained from the amplitudes of recovery tails (points 1–4). (Tsien 1970.) (b) Activation curve obtained by same technique in another preparation. (c) Rate coefficients of activation α_s and deactivation β_s as functions of membrane potential obtained from same fibre as (b). (Noble and Tsien 1968.)

range. This is shown in Fig. 7.3, where the activation curve is plotted. The activation variable chosen for this system was s, since it was the first of the slow K^+ currents to be analysed. For the same reason the current carried by the s channels was called $i_{K^+, 2}$ since it was thought to

93

correspond to the system similarly labelled i_{K2} in Hall, Hutter, and Noble's (1963) work and in the 1962 model. The current flow is therefore described by the equations (cf. eqns (2.5) and (2.7)),

$$i_{K^+_2} = \bar{i}_{K^+_2} \cdot s \tag{7.1}$$

$$\frac{ds}{dt} = \alpha_s(1 - s) - \beta_s s, \tag{7.2}$$

where $\bar{i}_{K^+_2}$ is the current carried by the channels when fully activated (see Fig. 7.5), α_s is the opening rate coefficient of the gating process, and β_s is the closing rate coefficient (cf. Fig. 2.3, p. 23).

This description of the pacemaker current immediately raises three problems. First, the current cannot be identical to the component $i_{K^+_2}$ in the 1962 model. This component activates at potentials positive to -50 mV (see Fig. 2.6, p. 29), as shown by Hall, Hutter, and Noble's experiments, whereas the component described in Figs 7.2 and 7.3 activates at very much more negative potentials. The answer to this problem lies in the fact that there are two distinct voltage ranges in which slow K^+ current changes occur in Purkinje fibres. The component labelled i_{K^+2} in the 1962 model corresponds to the largely K^+ current i_x described in the previous chapter. This must also have been the component observed by Hall, Hutter, and Noble (1963). The current controlled by the gating parameter s was not found in their experiments since these were carried out in Na^+-deficient solutions. For reasons that are not yet clear, the currents shown in Fig. 7.2 are not recorded in the absence of sodium ions.

This takes us to the second difficulty. The fact that sodium ions are required might suggest that the outward current changes result from the inactivation of an inward Na^+ current rather than from the activation of an outward K^+ current. This possibility may, however, be excluded by the observation that the reversal potential lies at the potassium equilibrium potential (Deck and Trautwein 1964; Noble and Tsien 1968; Peper and Trautwein 1969). Fig. 7.4 shows the observed reversal potential as a function of the extracellular K^+ concentration. As expected from eqn (2.2) there is a linear relation between the reversal potential and the logarithm of the K^+ concentration with a slope equal to RT/F.

The third problem lies in the role of i_{K^+2} in repolarization. Since i_{K^+2} is activated by even very small depolarizations it must be activated during the action-potential plateau. This is confirmed by the fact that a depolarization to, say, 0 mV is followed by a decay tail similar to

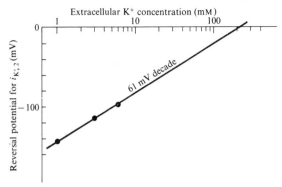

FIG. 7.4. Variation in reversal potential E_{K^+} for $i_{K^+, 2}$ as a function of log $[K^+]_0$. The straight line shows the relation given by the Nernst equation for E_{K^+} (eqn (2.2)). (Peper and Trautwein 1969.)

those shown in Fig. 7.2. Yet the onset of outward current at this potential is apparently fully accounted for by the activation of i_x as described in the previous chapter. This problem may be resolved by measuring the fully-activated current $\bar{i}_{K^+2}$, as a function of potential. The results of two experiments designed to do this are plotted in Fig. 7.5.

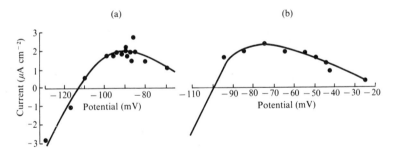

FIG. 7.5. Rectification displayed by the $i_{K^+, 2}$ channels in Purkinje fibres. (a) Current–voltage relation for $\bar{i}_{K^+, 2}$ (i.e. $i_{K^+, 2}$ when $s = 1$) (a) when $[K^+]_0 = 2$ mM. Reversal potential lies at -115 mV. (b) Relation in another fibre when $[K^+]_0 = 4$ mM. Reversal potential then lies at -100 mV. Note that current becomes small during strong depolarizations. This is the phenomenon of inward-going rectification (see Chapter 2, Fig. 2.2). (From Noble and Tsien (1968) and Hauswirth, Noble, and Tsien (1972b).)

Fig. 7.5(a) shows a curve obtained at $[K^+]_0 = 2$ mM in an experiment to determine the relation in the vicinity of the reversal potential. In this case, $E_{K^+} = -115$ mV (cf. Fig. 7.4). The current–voltage relation is

95

clearly very non-linear. Very much less current flows on depolarization than expected from a linear relation, and beyond -85 mV the relation displays a negative slope. The current at -70 mV is only about half that at -90 mV despite the larger driving force ($E_m - E_{K^+}$ is 45 mV at -70 mV and 25 mV at -90 mV). This is a striking example of the phenomenon of inward-going rectification (see p. 21).

Fig. 7.5(b) shows that the negative slope persists at large depolarizations so that, as the potential approaches 0, the current carried by the s channels becomes extremely small. Hence, even when fully-activated these channels contribute very little to the total repolarizing current. The largest current flow is carried in the pacemaker range of potentials.

Reconstruction of ionic current flow during pacemaker potential in Purkinje fibres

The next question, therefore, is whether the kinetics of the current flow in the pacemaker range are consistent with the view that $i_{K^+,2}$ controls the rate of pacemaker activity. We may answer this question by calculating how $i_{K^+,2}$ varies during the pacemaker potential.

First, we may note that during action potentials of normal duration s becomes fully activated. This is to be expected since the rate of activation (primarily determined by α_s) greatly increases on depolarization. Thus, at -60 mV the activation rate is much faster than at -75 mV (see Fig. 7.2). McAllister and Noble (1966) measured the activation time-constant at potentials in the plateau range and obtained a value of only 20 ms at -2 mV (see also Hauswirth, Noble, and Tsien 1972b). Thus s will become fully activated even during an action potential as short as 200 ms, which is the minimum duration approached at high frequencies (see Fig. 6.11, p. 88). We may assume therefore that at the beginning of the pacemaker potential $s = 1$ and $i_{K^+,2} = \bar{i}_{K^+,2}$. The steady-state value of s near -90 mV is 0 so that s will start to decay towards 0 at a rate determined by β_s at -90 mV (see Fig. 7.3), which is about 1 s^{-1} (i.e. a time-constant of 1 s). For example, during 0·1 s, s will decay by about 10 per cent, i.e. to 0·9, and $i_{K^+,2}$ will decay to 0·9 $\bar{i}_{K^+,2}$. As $i_{K^+,2}$ falls, the membrane will depolarize. The next steps must therefore be calculated with parameters of $\bar{i}_{K^+,2}$, α_s, and β_s appropriate to each potential. These are all known from the experimental results summarized in Figs 7.3 and 7.5.

The result of a calculation of this kind is shown in Fig. 7.6. The top diagram is a pacemaker potential recorded by Vassalle. The bottom diagram shows how s and $i_{K^+,2}$ vary with time. The first stages (up to

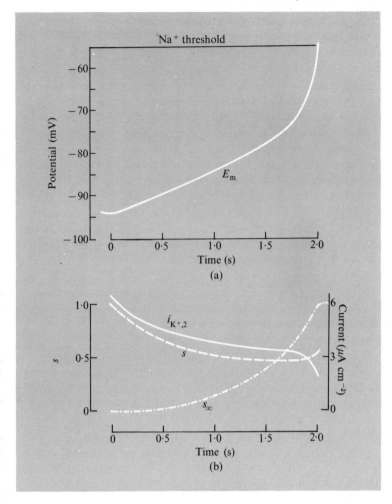

FIG. 7.6. Mechanism of Purkinje fibre pacemaker potential based on calculation using experimental data shown in Figs 7.4 and 7.5. (a) Variation of membrane potential during pacemaker depolarization (from Vassalle (1966). (b) Calculated changes in s and $i_{K^+,2}$ using eqns (7.1) and (7.2). The steady-state value s_∞ of the activation variable at each voltage is also plotted to show that s_∞ increases to equal the computed value of s at about 1·6 s. This is the point at which the change in s reverses direction. Beyond this time the continued depolarization depends on the fall in $\bar{i}_{K^+,2}$ (cf. Fig. 7.5) and on activation of i_{Na^+} when its threshold is approached. (Noble and Tsien 1968.)

about 1 s) are as expected from the calculation described above. s decays roughly exponentially at a rate of 10 per cent per 100 ms. Since $\bar{i}_{K^+,2}$ is nearly constant between -90 mV and -80 mV, $i_{K^+,2}$ also decays roughly exponentially. However, at potentials positive to -80 mV the calculation becomes more complex. First, the steady-state values s_∞ becomes appreciable (Fig. 7.3). This is the value that s tries to approach, so that, instead of decaying towards 0, s decays towards a larger value. The rate of decay therefore falls and, in particular, when s_∞ exceeds s (at 1·6 s) s must start to increase again.

This means that beyond 1·6 s the fraction of conducting channels *increases* with time. If $\bar{i}_{K^+2}$ were a linear function of potential, this would result in an *increase* in K^+ current and the pacemaker depolarization would cease. It is important therefore to ask why the depolarization continues beyond the time at which $s = s_\infty$. Part of the answer to this question lies in the fact that beyond -80 mV $\bar{i}_{K^+2}$ *decreases* with potential. Hence, despite the *increase* in the total number s of conducting channels, the current carried i_{K^+2} *decreases*. This is shown in Fig. 7.6. Beyond 1·6 s, the variables s and i_{K^+2} no longer follow similar time-courses. As s begins to increase, i_{K^+2} sharply falls. The terminal stage of the Purkinje-fibre pacemaker potential is thus dependent on the inward-rectifying property of the s channels.

A second factor that probably contributes to maintaining the depolarization when $s_\infty > s$ is that as the threshold is approached the Na^+ current begins to activate. During slow phases of potential change, when the net ionic current is exceedingly small, even a very small degree of Na^+ activation will increase the depolarization rate.

We may therefore regard the pacemaker potential as having two phases: an early phase (up to about 1·5 s in the case illustrated) which is primarily governed by the *time*-dependence of the decay of i_{K^+2}; and a late phase which is governed by the *voltage*-dependent decrease in $\bar{i}_{K^+2}$ and activation of i_{Na^+}.

Temperature-dependence of pacemaker current

One of the tests of this analysis of the pacemaker mechanism is to determine the way in which the rate coefficient β_s varies with temperature since, as shown in Fig. 7.1, the rate of depolarization is highly temperature-dependent. This requires either that the decay rate of the K^+ current should increase steeply with temperature or that the inward background current should increase with temperature. The latter seems unlikely since the result would be that the pacemaker potential would start at a more

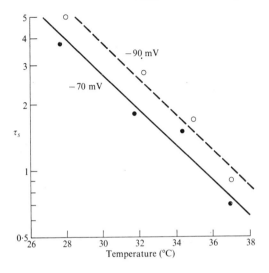

FIG. 7.7. Variation in τ_s with temperature. Log τ_s is plotted for two different potentials, $-70\,\text{mV}$ and $-90\,\text{mV}$ (o). The variation is roughly linear and the Q_{10} is 6 (cf. Fig. 7.1). (Noble and Tsien 1968.)

depolarized potential and so reach threshold more quickly. In fact the maximum negative potential at the beginning of the pacemaker depolarization becomes even more negative as the temperature is increased (Fig. 7.1).

Fig. 7.7 shows that the rate constants of the s reaction are highly temperature-dependent. The time-constant $\tau_s\,(\ = \ 1/(\alpha_s + \beta_s))$ was measured at two potentials (-70 mV and -90 mV) as the temperature was varied between 28 °C and 38 °C. At -90 mV the time-constant is virtually equal to $1/\beta_s$ since α_s is negligible (see Fig. 7.3). At -70 mV, α_s is also included. Any significant difference between the temperature-dependence of the rates of activation and decay therefore might be detected by this experiment. In fact the results are the same at both potentials. The time-constant decreases steeply with temperature. The lines show the decreases expected for a Q_{10} of 6. We may conclude therefore that the temperature-dependence of pacemaker activity shown in Fig. 7.1 is attributable to the high Q_{10} of the s rate constants.

Mechanism of pacemaker activity in atrial muscle

I have already referred to the substantial difference between the pacemaker range of potentials in the Purkinje fibre (-90 mV to -60 mV) and

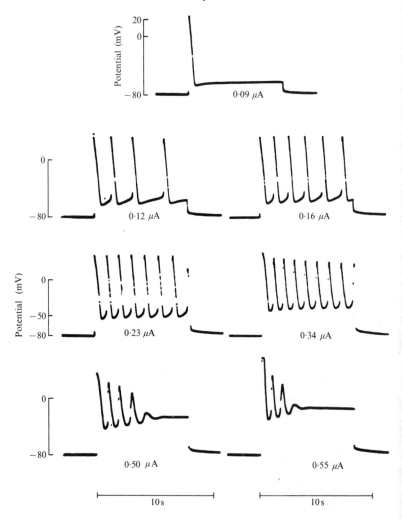

FIG. 7.8. Pacemaker responses of frog atrial trabeculum during application of small depolarizing currents (Brown and Noble 1969a).

in sinus and atrial tissue (-60 mV to -40 mV). At the very least this difference suggests caution in applying an analysis of one tissue to the other. Moreover, it is worth remembering that the Purkinje fibres do not normally generate the natural rhythm. Since the SA node fires at a higher frequency, the heart is normally driven by this region, and the

Purkinje fibres then act simply as a fast conducting system. Pacemaker activity in the Purkinje fibres is therefore important only in clinical conditions such as AV block, when the ventricles are driven at the relatively slow rate generated by the Purkinje fibres.

As yet it has proved difficult to perform voltage-clamp experiments on the SA node itself, although some preliminary analysis showing the presence of a pacemaker K^+ current has been described by Irisawa (1972). However, Brown and Noble (1969a) and Lenfant, Mironneau, and Aka (1972) have shown that normally quiescent atrial fibres may be induced to show pacemaker activity like that of the SA node simply by applying a steady depolarizing current. This is illustrated in Fig. 7.8, which shows the responses to various magnitudes of depolarizing current applied to a frog atrial trabeculum. The fibre was initially quiescent at a resting potential of -80 mV. The application of a current equal to $0.09\,\mu A$ produces a single action potential followed by a small, maintained depolarization that lasts as long as the applied current. Increasing the applied current to $0.12\,\mu A$ induces repetitive firing at a relatively low frequency. The frequency increases with the strength of the current up to $0.34\,\mu A$. Larger currents ($0.50\,\mu A$ and $0.55\,\mu A$) produced damped oscillations.

Notice that the maximum negative potential during induced pacemaker activity is only about -50 mV (see calibration on response to $0.23\,\mu A$), which is similar to records from the SA node and sinus (Fig. 1.3(a), p. 7).

The current changes underlying the pacemaker potential in this case were analysed as shown in Fig. 7.9. Following the application of the depolarizing current, the membrane was clamped at various potentials immediately after repolarization had occurred. The normal train of action potentials was therefore suppressed. The record showing three action potentials is part of a normal train of responses which is included to illustrate what would have happened in each case if the voltage clamp had not been applied. The other records are superimposed and show the results of clamping the membrane to four different potentials. At -40 mV and -60 mV, the current record is a decaying outward current. At -84 mV a decaying inward current is obtained. At -73 mV, which is close to the resting potential, the current record is level. This potential is therefore the reversal potential of the current mechanism responsible for pacemaker activity. Estimates of the K^+ equilibrium potential (Haas, Glitsch, and Kern 1966) suggest that it is about 20 mV negative to the resting potential. The pacemaker current in this preparation therefore resembles i_x rather than i_{K^+2} (see also Lenfant et. al. 1972).

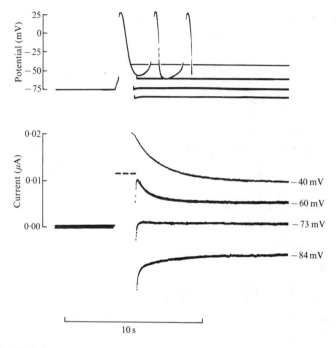

FIG. 7.9. Voltage-clamp analysis of pacemaker current in frog atrium. The clamp was applied at the end of the first action potential in each train. Outward current is shown as an upward deflection (Brown, Clark, and Noble 1972).

Further evidence for this view is provided by measuring activation curves for K^+ currents in atrial muscle. The threshold for activation is found to be about -40 mV (Rougier, Vassort, and Stämpfli 1968; Brown and Noble 1969a, b; Hemptinne 1971a) which is similar to the threshold for i_x in Purkinje fibres. Substantial currents in the s range (-90 mV to -60 mV) are not observed. It appears therefore that the s system is confined to Purkinje fibres since experiments on ventricular muscle also show no evidence of slow K^+ currents in the s range.

Thus, the pacemaker K^+ current in atrial muscle is not the same component as that in Purkinje fibres. Further differences between the two pacemaker mechanisms will be discussed in the next chapter.

8 Chronotropic actions of autonomic nervous transmitters

Although the beating of the heart is initiated by electrical changes occurring entirely within the heart, the frequency of beating is controlled by the nervous and hormonal systems. Vagal (parasympathetic) activity slows the rate, whereas sympathetic activity increases it. The chronotropic actions of the sympathetic and parasympathetic nervous systems are thus opposite. By itself this observation might suggest that the transmitters have opposing actions on one or other of the components of ionic current. We shall see in this chapter that this simple view is far from correct. The changes in ionic current produced by the parasympathetic transmitter (acetylcholine) are not generally reversed by the sympathetic transmitter (adrenaline).[†] An indication of the substantial difference between the mechanisms involved is given by the fact that the action of acetylcholine was determined long before the introduction of the voltage-clamp technique (Hutter 1957), whereas that of adrenaline has required this technique for its elucidation.

Early work on chronotropic mechanisms

Some of the important observations on the actions of vagus and sympathetic-nerve stimulation on the heart were made towards the end of the nineteenth century and in the early part of this century. Hutter (1957) has described this work in a valuable review on autonomic transmitters, and I am indebted to this review for the references to early work given in this chapter.

Nineteenth-century physiologists did not, of course, have direct intracellular recording techniques. However, they were able to obtain an indirect estimate of membrane-potential changes by recording the potential between injured and intact regions of muscle. At the cut region the cell potential is reduced to zero and current flows through the injury driven by the cell membrane potential in intact regions. The

---

[†] Although recent work by Giles and Tsien (1975) suggests that acetylcholine has an opposite action on $i_{Ca^{2+}}$ to that of adrenaline.

magnitude of this injury current and, hence, of the extracellular potential between the injured and uninjured regions is proportional to the magnitude of the membrane potential in the intact region. It is thus possible to record resting and action potentials using extracellular electrodes, although the records obtained are smaller than those obtained directly with intracellular electrodes. A technique of this kind was used by Burdon-Sanderson and Page (1883) to demonstrate the long duration of cardiac action potentials (the 'intracellular' records of action potentials in the tortoise heart shown in Fig. 1.5 (p. 11) were obtained using a modification of the technique).

Gaskell (1886, 1887) also used the method to make the important discovery that the resting potential of quiescent tortoise auricle is made more negative (i.e. the membrane is hyperpolarized) by stimulating the vagus and is reduced by stimulating the sympathetic nerve. Although the hyperpolarizing action of the vagus was confirmed by others (Samojloff 1914; Bayliss 1913; Monnier and Dubuisson 1934), Gaskell's work was not generally accepted, partly because a hyperpolarization is not observed under all conditions (e.g. Gotch 1887) and partly because it was thought by some to be artefactual. The importance of checking this point when intracellular electrodes became available was quickly appreciated and in 1953 Burgen and Terroux showed that acetylcholine does indeed produce a hyperpolarization in auricular fibres from the cat. They also suggested that the effect may be attributed to an increase in permeability to potassium ions.

Early work on the effects of sympathetic stimulation also appeared a little confusing and cast some doubt on the general validity of Gaskell's work. The depolarization he recorded in tortoise auricle was also found in the sinus venosus of the frog that had been inhibited by vagal stimulation (del Castillo and Katz 1955), but in strips of dog auricle Dudel and Trautwein (1956) found a substantial hyperpolarization produced by adrenaline. I shall discuss a possible explanation for this difference later in the chapter (p. 116).

Mechanism of action of acetylcholine

I have already stressed the importance of being cautious about applying results from one cardiac preparation to another region of the heart. The action of the vagus on quiescent auricle need not be the same as the action on the natural pacemaker in the SA node or sinus venosus. However, in this case, the comparison has turned out to be justified. Experiments on the sinus venosus of frog and tortoise and on the SA node of rabbits have shown that vagal stimulation produces **hyperpolarization** (del Castillo and Katz 1955; Hutter and Trautwein 1955, 1956; West 1955). Fig. 8.1 shows a result obtained from the frog sinus venosus.

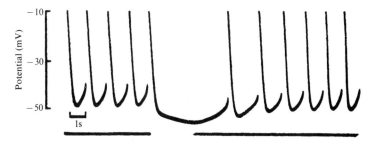

FIG. 8.1. Membrane potentials recorded in frog sinus venosus during vagus nerve stimulation (indicated by interruption in horizontal line). (Hutter and Trautwein 1956.)

During vagal stimulation the membrane hyperpolarizes by nearly 10 mV and pacemaker activity is suppressed. The hypothesis that this is attributable to an increase in K^+ permeability is supported by the observation that the membrane conductance is substantially increased (Trautwein, Kuffler, and Edwards 1956).

However, the most direct way of testing the hypothesis is to measure the K^+ movement across the membrane by using radioactive $^{42}K^+$. The result of such an experiment is shown in Fig. 8.2. A frog sinus venosus was 'loaded' with radioactive K^+ by incubating it for a period in radioactive solution. The preparation was then washed with non-radioactive solution, and the decrease in radioactivity with time was measured. The rate of decrease is a measure of the membrane permeability. During the period indicated the vagus nerve was stimulated at a rate of 10 impulses per second. The result is a large increase in the rate of loss of $^{42}K^+$ from the cells.

We may conclude therefore that the inhibitory action of acetylcholine is produced by a large increase in membrane K^+ conductance. In addition to slowing or abolishing pacemaker activity this would be expected to reduce the duration of the action potential by increasing the magnitude of the net repolarizing current. This is indeed the case. As shown in Fig. 8.3 the effect is so large that during the strongest inhibition it is impossible to initiate a propagated action potential. This effect on the action potential and its propagation is probably responsible for two

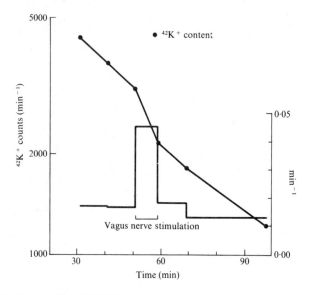

FIG. 8.2. Rate of efflux of $^{42}K^+$ in frog sinus venosus. Note more rapid loss of K^+ during period of vagus nerve stimulation (10 pulses per second) (Harris and Hutter, from Hutter 1961).

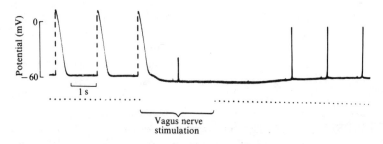

FIG. 8.3. Suppression of conducted action potentials in tortoise sinus venosus during stimulation of vagus nerve, indicated by interruption in dotted line. (Hutter and Trautwein 1956.)

other important effects of acetylcholine. First, the reduction in action-potential duration will result in a reduced amplitude and duration of contraction, i.e. acetylcholine has a negative inotropic action. Secondly, strong vagal stimulation can produce block of conduction at the AV node and so prevent atrial excitation spreading to the ventricle.

Actions of adrenaline on pacemaker cells

Despite the fact that pacemaker activity in sino-atrial tissue and in Purkinje fibres occurs at different potential ranges, the observed effect of adrenaline is very similar. As shown in Fig. 8.4 the major effect is an

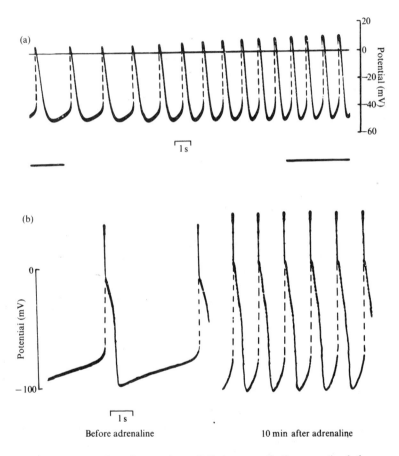

FIG. 8.4. Acceleration of pacemaker activity by sympathetic nerve stimulation and by adrenaline. (a) Frog sinus venosus. The sympathetic nerve was stimulated during break in horizontal line. (Hutter and Trautwein 1956.) (b) Sheep Purkinje fibre before and after application of adrenaline (Otsuka 1958).

acceleration of the rate of depolarization. It is also worth noting that in both cases the maximum negative potential at the end of the action potential is increased by adrenaline or by sympathetic nerve stimulation.

This hyperpolarization recalls Dudel and Trautwein's (1956) observation that the resting potential of dog auricle is increased by adrenaline, and it poses the dilemma that adrenaline both increases the depolarization rate and changes the peak negative potential to more hyperpolarized levels. It is difficult to see how a simple change in a single conductance can produce *both* of these effects. This suggests that we may be dealing with more than one action of adrenaline.

As I have already noted, the situation is not always as complex as this and Gaskell's (1887) observation that in quiescent tortoise auricle vagal and sympathetic nerve stimulation change the membrane potential in opposite directions suggests one possible explanation of the action of adrenaline: that it changes the membrane permeability to potassium ions in the opposite direction to that produced by acetylcholine. Attempts to demonstrate a decrease in $^{42}K^+$ efflux with adrenaline have however failed (Hutter 1957). Moreover, adrenaline has no marked effect on the resting membrane conductance nor does it influence the excitatory Na^+ conductance (Trautwein and Schmidt 1960; Kassebaum 1964). These observations also exclude another simple possibility: that adrenaline accelerates the depolarization during pacemaker activity by increasing the Na^+ current.

The mechanism of adrenaline action thus does not yield to the methods used so successfully to determine the mechanism of action of acetylcholine. When voltage-clamp techniques became available, therefore, it seemed important to see whether they would be more useful. This has proved to be the case. However, despite the similarity of the effects shown in Fig. 8.4, the ionic mechanisms of the action on Purkinje and atrial tissues have been found to be quite different (see Brown, McNaughton, Noble, and Noble 1975) and I shall deal with them separately.

Voltage-clamp analysis of adrenaline action in Purkinje fibres

A possible explanation for the increased depolarization rate in Purkinje fibres was suggested by the discovery that pacemaker activity in this preparation is controlled by a K^+ current i_{K^+2} activated at very negative potentials (see Chapter 7). It may help the reader to describe first the theoretical basis of this possible mechanism for the action of adrenaline before describing experiments designed to test it.

As shown in the previous chapter (see Fig. 7.6, p. 97) the rate of depolarization during the pacemaker potential is determined largely by the rate of decay of K^+ conductance, in turn determined by the decay of the gating variable s. At any given potential s decays following the equation

$$s = s_\infty - (s_\infty - s_0) \exp\{-(\alpha_s + \beta_s)\, t\}, \qquad (8.1)$$

where s_0 is the initial value of s. Moreover, as noted earlier (p. 96), at the beginning of the pacemaker potential (at around -90 mV) $s_0 = 1$ and α_s is negligible. Hence

$$s = s_\infty - (s_\infty - 1) \exp(-\beta_s t) \qquad (8.2)$$

and

$$ds/dt = -\beta_s (1 - s_\infty) \exp(-\beta_s t); \qquad (8.3)$$

so that to increase the rate of decay of s we must decrease s_∞ (so that $1 - s_\infty$ approaches its maximum value, i.e. 1) or increase β_s. Both effects may be produced by the simple device of shifting the α and β functions (and hence also s_∞ since $s_\infty = \alpha_s/(\alpha_s + \beta_s)$; see eqn (2.6), p. 23) on the voltage axis in a positive direction. This kind of shift may be produced in excitable cells by agents that change the **membrane** surface charge since this has the effect of changing the field within the membrane to which the gating reactions respond. Thus, in nerve fibres, hydrogen and calcium ions shift the Na^+ and K^+ current thresholds, presumably by neutralizing surface negative charge (see Hille 1968; Gilbert and Ehrenstein 1969).

The changes that such a shift in the s activation curve would produce on $i_{K^+,2}$ are illustrated diagrammatically in Fig. 8.5. The continuous curves represent the state of affairs before the shift; the interrupted curves represent the state of affairs after the shift. Before the shift we suppose that the decay of s is measured at about -80 mV as occurring from the point A to the point B. As shown in the lower diagram the change will be exponential and the rate of decay will be determined by the time-constant $(= 1/(\alpha_s + \beta_s))$ and the total magnitude of the change.

After the shift, the decay occurs from A to C. Even if there were no change in time constant the *absolute* rate of decay would be increased since the total amplitude of the decay is larger. This is shown by the interrupted decay curve. In fact, however, β_s is increased and the time-constant of decay is reduced. The decay from A to C therefore follows the much faster time-course given by the dotted curve.

A shift of this kind can readily be detected in voltage-clamp experiments. If we hold the membrane at about -80 mV, we would expect to find (a) a change in the steady-state current at the holding potential in the inward direction since the steady-state value of s, and hence, of $i_{K^+,2}$ is reduced; (b) a larger change in s on depolarizing the membrane; and

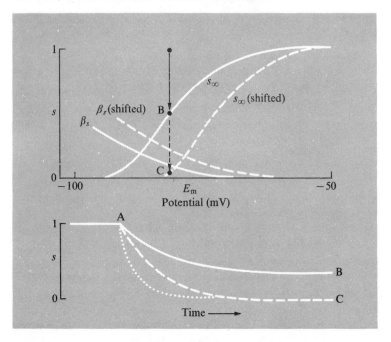

FIG. 8.5. Diagram illustrating possible mechanism of acceleration of pacemaker activity by adrenaline (Noble 1974).

(c) a smaller change in s on hyperpolarizing the membrane.

Fig. 8.6 shows the result of a voltage-clamp experiment on Purkinje fibre by Hauswirth, Noble, and Tsien (1968). The current record shown in Fig. 8.6(a) shows all three changes. The steady level of current at the holding potential (-80 mV) shifts in a negative (inward) direction; the recovery tail following a depolarization to -50 mV increases while the recovery tail following hyperpolarization to -90 mV is abolished. This means that the threshold for activation of i_{K^+2} must have shifted from its normal value of about -90 mV to a potential positive to -80 mV. Fig. 8.6(b) shows the activation curves obtained in this experiment. Adrenaline shifts the s_∞ curve by about 30 mV. The results also show that the β-blocker pronethalol can completely reverse the effect as expected since the chronotropic action of adrenaline on the heart is classified as a β action. For further details of the actions of adrenaline on i_{K^+2} the reader is referred to Tsien (1974a, b).

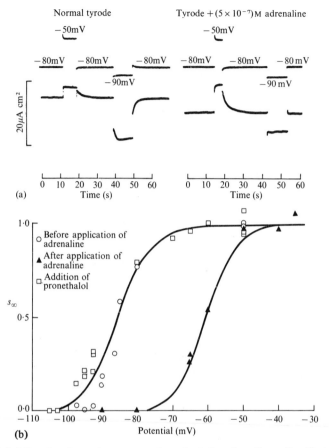

FIG. 8.6. Results of experiment to test hypothesis for adrenaline action illustrated in Fig. 8.5. (a) Current records in response to depolarizing and hyperpolarizing steps before (*left*) and after (*right*) application of adrenaline. (b) Activation curves before and after application of adrenaline. The effect is reversed by adding the β-blocker pronethalol. (Replotted from Hauswirth, Noble, and Tsien 1968.)

Reconstruction of chronotropic action of adrenaline

It is clear from Fig. 8.5 that a depolarizing shift in the *s* curve will accelerate the decay of *s* at negative potentials. The remaining question is whether this acceleration is sufficient to account for the chronotropic actions of adrenaline on Purkinje fibres. This question has been answered by incorporating various amounts of *s* shift in calculations of the pacemaker potential using a model of the ionic currents (Hauswirth,

Chronotropic actions of autonomic nervous transmitters

McAllister, Noble, and Tsien 1969; McAllister, Noble, and Tsien 1975). The results are shown in Fig. 8.7. Even relatively small potential shifts

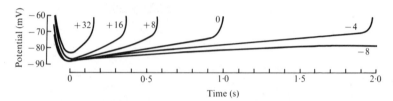

FIG. 8.7. Computed pacemaker potentials showing acceleration produced by voltage shifts in activation curve (McAllister, Noble, and Tsien 1975).

produce large changes in frequency. Thus a shift of 5 mV is sufficient to reduce the duration of the pacemaker potential by about 40 per cent. This diagram also shows that a small hyperpolarizing shift is adequate to suppress pacemaker activity. This effect is relevant to the observation that adrenaline will induce spontaneous activity in quiescent fibres. Thus a 4 mV depolarizing shift from the sixth case (which is quiescent) in Fig. 8.7 would be sufficient to induce pacemaker activity. We may conclude therefore that the shift in the s curve is adequate to account for the increased frequency produced by adrenaline.

However, there is one important respect in which the results calculated in Fig. 8.7 do not reproduce the experimental results shown in Fig. 8.4(b). This is that in the calculated responses the maximum negative potential is *reduced* by adrenaline, whereas experimentally it is found to increase in Purkinje fibres. This effect must be additional to the action on i_{K_2}. One possibility is that it is attributable to stimulation of the $Na^+ - K^+$ exchange pump which is known to occur in the presence of adrenaline (Vassalle and Barnabei 1971). This activation would have the effect of increasing the K^+ concentration gradient so that E_{K^+} would become more negative. Moreover, if the pump does carry a net hyperpolarizing current (see p. 17) a direct contribution to the maximum negative potential would be expected.

Finally, it is important to ask why the early attempts to measure K^+ conductance changes during adrenaline action failed. Part of the answer lies in the fact that the reduction in steady-state K^+ conductance occurs only over the very narrow voltage range of the s activation curve. Moreover since this curve is steeply dependent on voltage, the potential changes produced would tend to counter the primary effect. Thus, a reduction of

$i_{K^+_2}$ due to a depolarizing shift would tend to depolarize the membrane which in turn leads to reactivation of $i_{K^+_2}$. During spontaneous activity the situation is even more complex. Although under the influence of adrenaline $i_{K^+_2}$ decays *towards* a lower steady-state value, it has less time to approach this value since the duration of the pacemaker depolarization is reduced. The *average* K$^+$ conductance, and K$^+$ fluxes, may therefore remain unchanged by adrenaline. There is only one kind of experiment that should unambiguously reveal a decrease in K$^+$ efflux. This is to measure the K$^+$ efflux in a voltage-clamped Purkinje fibre whose potential is held constant at, say -75 mV. During a $15-20$ mV shift in s, s_∞ should decrease from 0·5 to 0. Since $i_{K^+_2}$ contributes about 50 per cent of the total K$^+$ conductance in the pacemaker range (the remainder being attributable to $i_{K^+_1}$ —see Chapter 9) we would expect a decrease in K$^+$ flux of the order of 25 per cent in such an experiment. So far, it has not been possible to perform this experiment since the ^{42}K$^+$ fluxes from the short segment of Purkinje fibre required for voltage-clamp analysis are very small.

Voltage-clamp analysis of adrenaline action in atrial fibres

In the previous chapter I described the evidence that pacemaker activity in atrial muscle is controlled by a K$^+$ current resembling $i_{x,1}$ rather than $i_{K^+_2}$. The activation curves and ionic selectivities of these two components are markedly different. Moreover, in Purkinje fibres the action of adrenaline on i_x (see p. 87) is very different from the action on $i_{K^+, 2}$ described above. It is therefore important to determine whether the mechanism of acceleration of atrial pacemaker activity by adrenaline is similar to that in Purkinje fibres. Experiments to achieve this aim have been performed recently by H.F. Brown and S.J. Noble. Fig. 8.8 shows one of their results. The records shown in Fig. 8.8(a) are repetitive responses to the same applied depolarizing current before and after applying adrenaline. Two major changes are observed. The action-potential height is increased and the pacemaker activity occurs at a more negative range of potentials. The 'threshold' for induced pacemaker activity thus becomes more negative and a smaller depolarization is required to initiate an action potential.

Fig. 8.8(b) shows the activation curves for the K$^+$ current i_x before and after applying adrenaline. The result is strikingly different from that obtained on the $i_{K^+_2}$ activation curve in Purkinje fibres (Fig. 8.6). There is no depolarizing shift and there is a marked increase in the amplitude of the current flow. The increase in amplitude of i_x with adrenaline is also seen in Purkinje fibres (see p. 87). However, the negative-going shift in

Chronotropic actions of autonomic nervous transmitters

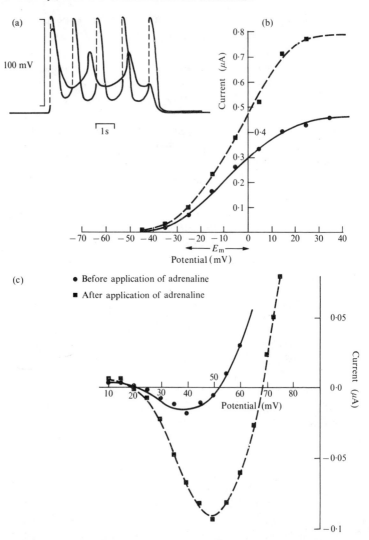

FIG. 8.8. Actions of adrenaline (5×10^{-9} M) on atrial pacemaker activity and ionic currents involved. (a) Pacemaker responses to small depolarizing current before and after application of adrenaline. (b) Increase in amplitude of K⁺ current, i_x, by application of adrenaline. (c) Effect of adrenaline on inward Ca^{2+} current. (Brown and Noble 1974.)

threshold which is observed in Purkinje fibres (Tsien, Giles, and Greengard 1972) does not appear to occur in the atrium.

As already noted in a previous chapter (p. 88) an increase in amplitude of i_x will reduce the action-potential duration, or at least prevent its prolongation by the accompanying increase in Ca^{2+} current. The effect on pacemaker activity, however, should be to slow the rate since a larger activation of K^+ current during the action potential will ensure that repolarization occurs to a more negative potential (as is observed in Fig. 8.8(a)) and the larger decrease in i_x necessary for the pacemaker depolarization to reach firing threshold should take longer to occur. Thus, the K^+ current changes induced in atrial fibres by adrenaline are precisely opposite to those required in order to accelerate the rate of beating. The observed acceleration must therefore be attributed to an action on another ionic current. The obvious candidate is the Ca^{2+} current which is known to be increased by adrenaline (see p. 67). In Purkinje fibres the pacemaker potential occurs at potentials largely negative to the Ca^{2+} threshold but in atrial and sinus tissue the more positive range at which the pacemaker potential occurs means that it may be influenced by the magnitude of the Ca^{2+} current (Lenfant, Mironneau, and Aka 1972; Brooks and Lu 1972). Fig. 8.8(c) shows the increase in Ca^{2+} current produced by adrenaline.

To the extent that pacemaker activity in the SA node resembles that induced in atrial fibres rather than that in Purkinje fibres it seems probable that the actions of adrenaline on SA pacemaker activity are also attributable to increases in $i_{Ca^{2+}}$ and i_x. If this is so, the resemblances in the records shown in Fig. 8.4 must be superficial. The increase in the rate of pacemaker depolarization is produced by an increased rate of decay of $i_{K^+_2}$ in Purkinje fibres but probably by an increase in $i_{Ca^{2+}}$ in SA fibres. The increased negativity of the peak diastolic potential may also be produced by different mechanisms. An increased activation of i_x during the action potential may be responsible for the repolarization to a more negative potential in SA and atrial tissue. In Purkinje fibres, although the activation of i_x is increased, it is less certain to produce the increased membrane potential following repolarization since the reversal potential for i_x is not usually sufficiently negative.

Summary of the actions of adrenaline

Clearly we have advanced considerably in elucidating the mechanisms of action of adrenaline since Hutter's review of 1957. However, his conclusion that 'at the moment it is therefore difficult to discuss the action of adrenaline in general terms' is still true. The elucidation of the actions of adrenaline using voltage-clamp techniques has not enabled us to produce a single primary cause comparable to the K^+ permeability change produced by acetylcholine. Instead we have a somewhat disparate set of effects and do not yet know whether they have any common cause other than that they are all produced by adrenaline. Since I have discussed these various effects in different chapters it may help the reader briefly to summarize them and their role in mediating the known inotropic and chronotropic actions of adrenaline.

1. The Ca^{2+} current is substantially increased. This effect is responsible for the increased height of the action potential, probably for the positive inotropic action and for the increased pacemaker rate in sino-atrial and atrial tissue.

2. The activation curve for $i_{K^+_2}$ in Purkinje fibres is shifted in a depolarizing direction. This effect is responsible for the acceleration of pacemaker activity in Purkinje fibres.

3. The K^+ current i_x is increased in amplitude and, in some cases, its activation threshold is reduced. This effect is responsible for shortening the action potential and, in SA and atrial tissue, for increasing the maximum negative potential in diastole.

4. The activity of the Na^+–K^+ exchange pump is increased. This effect may be responsible for the increased maximum negative potential in diastole in Purkinje fibres.

It is worth asking whether, in the light of these known actions, we may account for the puzzling difference between Gaskell's (1887) and del Castillo and Katz's (1955) observations that adrenaline may depolarize a quiescent membrane and Dudel and Trautwein's (1956) observation that a marked hyperpolarization may occur. It is plausible to suggest that whether depolarization or hyperpolarization is obtained may depend on how close the membrane potential is to the Ca^{2+} current threshold. If it is close to this threshold, the increase in Ca^{2+} current may predominate and lead to depolarization. At more negative membrane potentials the Ca^{2+} current will be negligible and the hyperpolarizing influence of the Na^+–K^+ pump may be important. It is too early to say whether this explanation is correct but it is at least clear now that both depolarizing and hyperpolarizing effects of adrenaline are consistent with the known actions of adrenaline.

Finally, I shall conclude this chapter by noting a further remarkable difference between the action of acetylcholine and all the known actions of adrenaline. Acetylcholine affects a purely passive conductance that simply produces an increase in K^+ current flow at all potentials. In this respect its action is similar to that of transmitters at many other synapses.

By contrast, the cardiac actions of adrenaline are all on membrane mechanisms that are 'active', either in the sense that they are Hodgkin–Huxley -type conductances producing K^+ or Ca^{2+} currents that are highly dependent on the membrane potential, or that they are energy-consuming, like the Na^+ pump.

9 Background currents and the effects of plasma ion concentration

In previous chapters I have discussed the properties and functions of the Na^+, Ca^{2+}, and K^+ currents that are activated and inactivated by membrane-potential changes. These currents are functions not only of voltage but also of time since the activation and inactivation processes take time to occur. There are also currents that display no significant time dependence and these currents are functionally important in cardiac muscle. Thus, the K^+ current i_{K^+1} used in the 1962 model (Fig. 2.6, p. 29) is voltage-dependent only and plays a large role in repolarization.

In their analysis of nerve membrane currents in 1952, Hodgkin and Huxley found a component remaining when the voltage- and time-dependent Na^+ and K^+ currents were allowed for. They called this current the 'leak' current since it represents those ions that leak through the membrane other than through the channels controlled by the m, h, and n gating mechanisms. The term 'leak current' is often used in another sense in cardiac electrophysiology: to refer to current leaking through damaged regions following dissection or through the sucrose solutions of a sucrose-gap system (see Chapter 3). It is therefore preferable to use another term for genuine membrane currents that remain when all the time-dependent currents have been accounted for. Since time-independent currents are present throughout a sequence of voltage changes and determine the 'background' level of current flow on which the time-dependent currents are superimposed, I shall refer to them as 'background' currents.

In nerve membrane the background current i_1 is very small compared to the net currents flowing during depolarization and repolarization. In cardiac muscle, by contrast, the net repolarizing current is very small (see Chapter 6) and the background current may then contribute a large fraction of the repolarizing current (Hemptinne 1971b).

In this chapter I shall describe two components of background current, outward and inward, although this does not necessarily imply the existence of separate membrane channels for the two components.

The background K⁺ current

The outward component corresponds to the outward K^+ current i_{K^+1} that may be recorded below the threshold for time-dependent K^+ currents. In atrial and ventricular fibres this threshold lies at or beyond -40 mV so that i_{K^+1} may be measured with little interference from i_x up to this potential. When the activation range for i_x is entered, $i_{K^+,1}$ may still be estimated from the *initial* magnitude of the outward current before i_x has had time to activate (see Fig. 9.1). Experiments of this

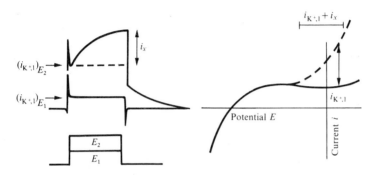

FIG. 9.1. Illustration of how a net K^+-current record may be divided into time-independent ($i_{K^+,1}$) and time-dependent (in this case i_x) components.

kind are best performed in the absence of Na^+ and Ca^{2+} currents. These conditions may be achieved either by using selective blocking agents (tetrodotoxin and manganese ions — see p. 60) or by using ion-deficient solutions. In Purkinje fibres the situation is also complicated by the activation of the pacemaker K^+ current $i_{K^+,2}$ at potentials positive to -90 mV. In this case the background currents may be calculated, once the kinetics of $i_{K^+,2}$ are known, by subtracting $i_{K^+,2}$ from the total current—voltage relation (see Hauswirth, Noble, and Tsien 1972b). Alternatively, experiments may be performed in Na^+-free solutions when current changes due to $i_{K^+,2}$ are absent and the threshold for time-dependent K^+ currents then lies at more depolarized potentials (McAllister and Noble 1966).

Whichever method is used, the result is the same in all cardiac fibres: the background K^+ current i_{K^+1} is a non-linear function of the membrane potential. The current recorded on depolarizing the membrane is much less than expected. This phenomenon is known as inward-going rectification and I have already discussed its functional importance in minimizing energy loss during cardiac electrical activity (see p. 74). In this chapter I shall discuss some additional properties of cardiac muscle that are attributable to inward-going rectification.

First, however, it is worth examining the evidence that this is genuine rectification displayed by the K^+ channels, rather than, for example, the addition of an inward background current during depolarization that reduces the net outward current. This may be tested by measuring the movement of radioactive $^{42}K^+$ as a function of the membrane potential. If the electrical rectification is attributable to K^+ current flow then the K^+ permeability, as measured by $^{42}K^+$ fluxes, should fall when the membrane is depolarized. An experiment of this kind was performed by Haas and Kern (1966) who measured the radioactive K^+ flux in a voltage-clamped Purkinje fibre in Na^+-free solution. They succeeded in showing that the current—voltage relation reconstructed from the flux measurements partly resembles that of the outward background current (see Fig. 9.2). This experiment confirms the view that most of

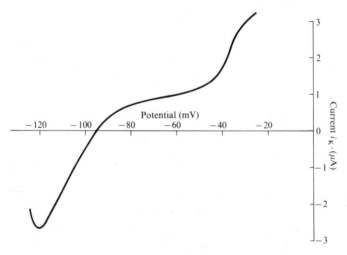

FIG. 9.2. Current-voltage diagram for $i_{K^+, 1}$ reconstructed from $^{42}K^+$ flux measurements (Haas and Kern 1966).

this current is carried by potassium ions and justifies the use of the symbol $i_{K^+_1}$ to identify it.

Background currents and the effects of plasma ion concentration

Electrogenic pump current

In most excitable cells the Na^+-K^+ exchange pump is electrogenic. It extrudes more Na^+ than it pumps K^+ into the cell and so carries a net outward current (see p. 17). This current may also contribute to the background outward current, as has been shown by Isenberg and Trautwein (1974) who used cardiac glycosides to block the Na^+ pump. They found that this decreases the background outward current by a significant amount at all potentials.

Inward background current

The presence of an inward background current may be deduced from the fact that the resting potential (between -80 mV and -90 mV) is not equal to the K^+ equilibrium potential (between -115 mV and -100 mV depending on whether the K^+ concentration outside the cell is taken as 2·7 or 4 mM). The magnitude of the inward current may be estimated by measuring the inward current required to hyperpolarize the membrane to the K^+ equilibrium potential (see Fig. 9.3). A fairly

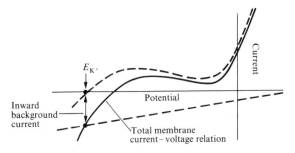

FIG. 9.3. Illustration of how the inward background current may be estimated from knowledge of total membrane current–voltage relation and of value of E_{K^+} obtained by measuring reversal potential for $i_{K^+, 2}$ (see Fig. 7.4).

substantial current is required to do this. Unfortunately, very little is known about this current. It is usually assumed to be a Na^+ current and that its current–voltage relation is linear. These were the assumptions made in the 1962 model. However, the cell membrane does not hyperpolarize to E_{K^+} in Na^+-free solutions (Draper and Weidmann 1951; Dudel et al. 1966), although a partial hyperpolarization is sometimes recorded (see e.g. Hall, Hutter, and Noble 1963). It is possible, of course, that substitutes for Na^+, such as choline, may also pass through the channels conducting the inward background current. A significant choline permeability has been found in cardiac muscle (Bosteels, Vleugels, and Carmeliet 1970).

The function of the inward background current is important not only in determining the resting potential by depolarizing the membrane to a potential positive to E_{K^+} but also in pacemaker activity. The decay of the K^+ currents $i_{K^+_2}$ and $i_{x,1}$ can only lead to pacemaker depolarization if a steady inward depolarizing current is also present.

The influence of extracellular potassium ions on the K^+ currents

The level of extracellular K^+ has a profound influence on electrical activity in cardiac muscle. Moreover, variations in plasma K^+ are important in clinical conditions associated with heart disease. Since many of the important effects of extracellular K^+ may be explained by studying the influence of K^+ on the inward-rectification shown by $i_{K^+_1}$ (Noble 1965) it is appropriate to discuss this topic in this chapter, both for its own sake as an illustration of the otherwise puzzling properties of cardiac muscle attributable to inward-going rectification, and for its clinical importance. In this section I shall show how $i_{K^+_1}$ is influenced by external potassium ions. The consequences of these effects for the electrical behaviour of the heart will be discussed in the next section.

One might expect that to increase the extracellular K^+ concentration would increase the influx of potassium ions from outside the cell and so reduce the net outflow of K^+ responsible for the measured K^+ current. This would reduce the net repolarizing current and so prolong the action potential duration. We should then find that potassium ions have a positive inotropic effect since the prolonged action potential would lead to a larger and stronger contraction. None of these expectations is fulfilled. The cardiac action potential is greatly shortened by increasing $[K^+]_0$ (Brooks, Hoffman, Suckling, and Orias 1955; Coraboeuf and Otsuka 1956; Weidmann 1956). A particularly striking example of this phenomenon was provided by Weidmann's experiment illustrated in Fig. 9.4 in which a turtle-heart action potential was shortened by injecting potassium ions via the coronary artery during the action potential plateau. Sidney Ringer (1883) had shown that K^+ has a negative inotropic action, i.e. reduces the strength of contraction. This may be partly attributed to the shortened action potential (see p. 129).

It appears then that extracellular potassium ions must increase the net repolarizing current. A possible explanation for this anomalous action

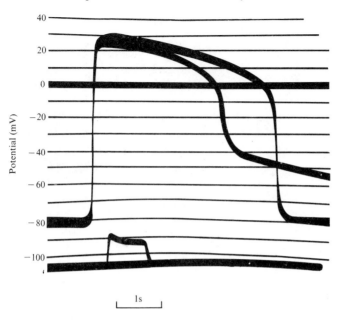

FIG. 9.4. Shortening of turtle ventricle action potential by injection of K$^+$ via coronary artery (Weidmann 1956).

may be provided by noting that an increase in the extracellular K$^+$ concentration shifts E_{K^+} in a positive direction and so reduces the net driving force $(E_m - E_{K^+})$ at any given potential. By itself this would reduce the K$^+$ current, since

$$i_{K^+} = g_{K^+} (E_m - E_{K^+}). \qquad (9.1)$$

However, if the fall in g_{K^+} on depolarization is determined by the magnitude of the driving force so that g_{K^+} is reduced when this force is large and outward, it is conceivable that a reduction in driving force may allow g_{K^+} to recover and so allow i_{K^+} to increase. An explanation of this kind was discussed by Hoffman and Cranefield (1960). A quantitative formulation was provided in Noble (1965) and an experimental test of the idea was performed by McAllister and Noble (1966).

We may illustrate the idea by using the function describing the inward-rectification shown by $i_{K^+_1}$ in the 1962 model. This is illustrated in Fig. 9.5 which also compares the model with a much simpler one that satisfies the expectations discussed at the beginning of this section. Fig. 9.5(a) shows the current–voltage diagrams that one would expect if

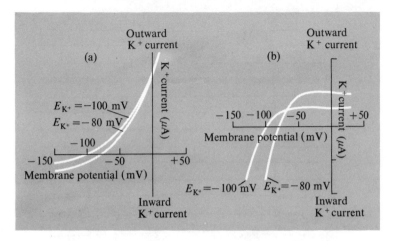

FIG. 9.5. Expected effects of increasing $[K^+]_0$ on K^+-current–voltage relations. (a) Assuming no inward-rectification. (b) When inward rectification is present. (Noble 1965.)

inward-rectification is absent. Curves for two values of E_{K^+} are plotted, -100 mV and -80 mV, with the K^+ permeability P_{K^+} constant (the equations used are the constant field equations described by Goldman (1943) and by Hodgkin and Katz (1949)). Note that, as expected, the outward current is always less at the higher extracellular concentration ($E_{K^+} = 80$ mV). The curves plotted in Fig. 9.5(b) were obtained by letting ($E_m - E_{K^+}$) be the parameter that determines the K^+ permeability such that P_{K^+} falls when ($E_m - E_{K^+}$) increases. The equation used is the same as that used for $i_{K^+_1}$ in the 1962 model (see Noble 1962a, 1965). The result is now quite different. The two relations intersect each other so that beyond the intersection point the K^+ current is always larger when the extracellular K^+ concentration is high. Fig. 9.6 shows the results of two experiments on Purkinje fibres in which the current–voltage relations were measured in Na^+-free solutions at two different K^+ concentrations, 4 mM and 24 mM. The results clearly resemble those of Fig. 9.5(b) rather than Fig. 9.5(a).

We may conclude therefore that an increase in K^+ concentration does increase the net outward current at potentials beyond the 'cross-over' voltage. Inward-going rectification is not only shown by $i_{K^+_1}$. It is also very marked in the case of $i_{K^+_2}$ (see Fig. 7.5, p. 95) and it is interesting to ask whether the 'cross-over' phenomenon is also shown. Experimental evidence that this is the case was provided by Noble and Tsien (1968).

124

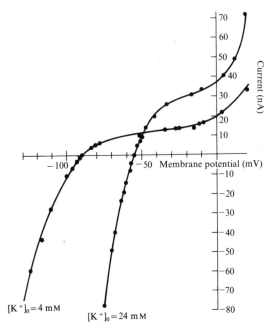

FIG. 9.6. Current–voltage diagrams for Purkinje fibres in Na⁺-free solutions in presence of 4 mM and 24 mM K⁺. Note resemblance to Fig. 9.5(b). (McAllister and Noble 1966.)

The phenomenon is also seen in the inward-rectifying K^+ channel in skeletal muscle (Adrian 1965). It appears therefore to be a property characteristic of ionic channels showing inward-going rectification.

The influence of potassium ions on action potential and pacemaker activity

We may now ask the question whether these effects are quantitatively adequate to explain the actions of potassium ions on action-potential duration and on pacemaker activity. Fig. 9.7 shows a comparison between experimental and computed effects of $[K^+]_0$ changes. The curves plotted in Fig. 9.7(a) were obtained using the 1962 model. Although this model is now replaced by a more accurate one (McAllister, Noble, and Tsien 1975) based on voltage-clamp experiments, there is no reason to expect that the effects of $[K^+]_0$ changes should be significantly different since the important effects are attributable to changes in $i_{K^+_1}$. The role played by this current is the same in the two models.

When $[K^+]_0$ is increased to shift E_{K^+} from -100 mV to -80 mV, a

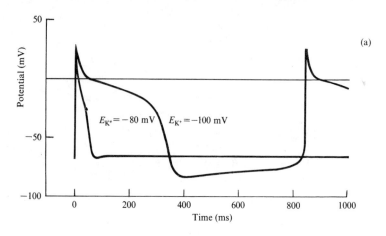

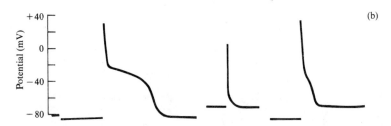

FIG. 9.7. Computed and observed effects of increasing $[K^+]_0$ on action potential and pacemaker activity. (a) Computed effects (Noble 1965). (b) Observed effects (Weidmann 1956) of normal (*left*) and three times normal (*centre* and *right*) $[K^+]$.

marked shortening of the action potential occurs and pacemaker activity is abolished. The records shown in Fig. 9.7(b) show the effects observed experimentally by Weidmann (1956). The fibre used by Weidmann was not a pacemaker fibre, but the abolition of pacemaker activity by increased $[K^+]_0$ does also occur experimentally in pacemaker fibres (Vassalle 1965).

The influence of potassium ions on the resting potential

The action of potassium ions on the resting potential in cardiac muscle is also found to be anomalous. Vaughan-Williams (1959) found that in rabbit atrial fibres the relative value of P_{K^+} compared to P_{Na^+} falls at low values of $[K^+]_0$ so that the resting potential is lower than expected. In Purkinje fibres, this effect is even more dramatic. As shown in Fig. 9.8(b),

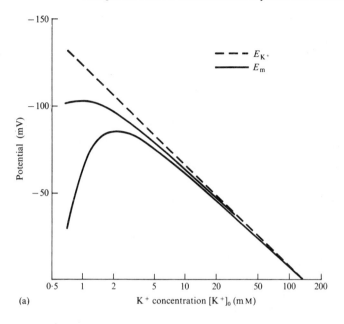

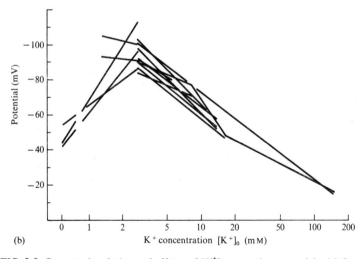

FIG. 9.8. Computed and observed effects of $[K^+]_0$ on resting potentials. (a) Computed effects assuming two different values (1 and 2) for g_{Na^+} at rest. *Lower curve:* $g_{Na^+} = 0.3 \text{ ms cm}^{-2}$; *middle curve:* $g_{Na^+} = 0.067 \text{ ms cm}^{-2}$ (Noble 1965). (b) Experimental relation in Purkinje fibre (Weidmann 1956).

127

the resting potential falls at low values of $[K^+]_0$. Similar values (-50 mV) of resting potential are obtained when $[K^+] = 20$ mM and when $[K^+]_0$ < 1 mM. However, the state of the membrane is very different in these two conditions. Depolarization at high values of $[K^+]_0$ is accompanied by an increase in membrane conductance, whereas depolarization at low values of $[K^+]_0$ is accompanied by a large decrease in membrane conductance (Carmeliet 1961). Carmeliet's observations, and the fact that sodium ions are required for the depolarization at low $[K^+]_0$ to occur, suggest a possible explanation. As $[K^+]_0$ is reduced, E_{K^+} becomes more negative. Since the membrane potential deviates most from E_{K^+} at low values of $[K^+]_0$ (this happens even if P_{K^+} and P_{Na^+} remain constant) the K^+ channels are subjected to an increasingly large outward driving force as $[K^+]_0$ is reduced. We should therefore expect the value of g_{K^+} to fall as a consequence of the presence of inward-going rectification. This would then allow the background Na^+ current to depolarize the membrane.

Fig. 9.8(a) shows the resting potential calculated as a function of $[K^+]_0$ using K^+ current—voltage diagrams given by the equations used for Fig. 9.5(b). The shape of the relation depends on the value of the background Na^+ conductance. When g_{Na^+} is set to the lower value (0.067 mS cm^{-2}) there is no significant depolarization at low $[K^+]_0$. This is similar to the situation in atrial and ventricular muscle. When g_{Na^+} is increased to 0.13 mS cm^{-2} the computed relation reproduces the Purkinje fibre results shown in Fig. 9.8(b).

Competition between extracellular K^+, Ca^{2+}, and Na^+

In addition to observing that potassium ions reduce the contractile response of cardiac muscle, Sidney Ringer (1883) also found that calcium ions increase it. He therefore concluded 'that the normal [tension] trace is the result of the antagonising action of calcium and potassium salts'. We may now give some explanation for this antagonism and compare it with that occurring between Na^+ and Ca^{2+}.

The dependence of cardiac contraction on extracellular calcium ions is very striking. At very low values of $[Ca^{2+}]_0$ the tension is reduced to zero despite the fact that action potentials still occur in response to electrical stimuli. This situation contrasts strongly with that in skeletal muscle where the dependence of contraction on extracellular Ca^{2+} is much less evident. As we have seen in Chapter 5, the strong dependence of cardiac contraction on extracellular Ca^{2+} is attributable to the fact that entry of calcium ions in the form of Ca^{2+} current during the action potential is an important step in the excitation—contraction coupling process. The strength of contraction is not simply related to the quantity of Ca^{2+} entering during each action potential (see Chapter 5, and review by Morad and Goldman (1973)) but there can be little doubt that this quantity is one of the factors determining the magnitude of contraction. The dependence of contraction on the duration of the action potential is thus attributable to the fact that the Ca^{2+}-current flow is dependent on the action-potential duration. If the membrane is repolarized very quickly, the Ca^{2+} current is turned off more rapidly. Part of the negative inotropic action of potassium ions may therefore be attributable to the reduction in action-potential duration discussed above. There is no need to postulate any direct competition between calcium and potassium ions at ion-binding or carrying sites on the membrane. (However, Morad and Goldman (1973) have recently proposed that such competition does nevertheless exist and that some Ca^{2+} entry is linked to K^+ outflow. It is too early to say whether this theory is correct.)

This situation contrasts sharply with the well-known competition between calcium and sodium ions (Lüttgau and Niedergerke 1958; Niedergerke 1963; Orkand and Niedergerke 1966). Here, there is a well-established stoichiometry in which two sodium ions appear to compete with one calcium ion. Thus the tension produced is dependent on the ratio $[Ca^{2+}]_0/[Na^+]_0^2$. These observations suggest that there is a membrane site which may bind either one calcium ion or two sodium ions. If this site were the one responsible for the selection of ions to be carried by the 'Ca^{2+}-current' mechanism then the entry of calcium ions would be dependent on the ratio $[Ca^{2+}]_0/[Na^+]_0^2$ and the negative inotropic effect of sodium ions would be attributable to a decrease in the fraction of the secondary inward current carried by calcium ions. As shown in Chapter 5, this current is not abolished when $[Ca^{2+}]_0$ is reduced to zero, which suggests that sodium ions may also be carried. In this context it is interesting to note that Rougier and Vassort (1971) have shown that the reversal potential for the secondary inward current in atrial muscle varies with extracellular ion concentrations in a way which is consistent with the view that the relative ion contributions to the current flow are determined by the ratio $[Ca^{2+}]_0/[Na^+]_0^2$.

The explanation for the positive inotropic effect of low-plasma K^+ is probably more complex. It may be due partly to an increase in action potential duration, but it is also possible that at sufficiently low values of $[K^+]_0$ the activity of the Na^+-K^+ exchange pump is reduced (see p. 16). This would allow the intracellular Na^+ concentration to increase and, in turn, we may also expect an increase in intracellular Ca^{2+} since the Na^+ and Ca^{2+} flows across the membrane are linked (see p. 17). Hence, at sufficiently low values of $[K^+]_0$ the intracellular Ca^{2+} stores might be increased. Whether this effect occurs and whether it contributes to the positive inotropic action is by no means certain but it is worth noting a possible resemblance here to the inotropic effects of the cardiac glycosides. These also reduce the activity of the Na^+ pump (see p. 17).

10 Abnormal electrical activity in the heart

Throughout this book I have referred to the medical importance of recent work on cardiac electrophysiology. Ideally, one would like to proceed to use the knowledge of the ionic currents we have acquired using new techniques to explain abnormal electrical activity and, perhaps, to suggest ways in which arrhythmias might best be treated. We are, however, still a long way from this goal. The mechanisms of arrhythmias and of fibrillation are still very unclear, and it is probable that a large number of factors are involved in the transformation from physiological to pathological states (see Surawicz 1971). In a short book of this kind one cannot possibly do justice to the very substantial body of important physiological, pharmacological, and clinical work that has been done in this field. Rather, I shall illustrate the way in which electrophysiology of the heart may be applied to clinical problems by singling out for discussion a few examples. These examples are largely restricted to problems that are easily related to earlier chapters, although the discussion is also more speculative than in the rest of the book.

Basis of continued rhythm during AV conduction block

First of all, it is important to note that the most serious common disturbances are ventricular. Atrial fibrillation, in which the atrial muscle fibres contract asynchronously and so cease to pump effectively, is not usually fatal unless accompanied by serious ventricular disorder. The ventricles are able to fill during diastole even without synchronized atrial contraction and so, provided the ventricles continue to beat, the heart may continue to pump blood into the arterial circulation. This is very strikingly illustrated by the fact that failure of conduction in the atrio-ventricular (AV) node is not fatal. The AV node is a region in which the action potentials are small and conduct very slowly (Mendez and Moe 1972), and a variety of factors (such as vagal stimulation − see p. 106) may produce failure to conduct since the safety factor for conduction is not very large. The auricular excitation then fails to spread to the ventricles and the P wave of the electrocardiogram (see Fig. 1.1, p. 3) is not followed in the usual way by the Q,R,S, and T waves. However, it is rare for the ventricles to stop beating (other than temporarily) in this situation. It is usually found that the ventricular components of the electrocardiogram appear regularly but at a lower frequency than the P waves. Sometimes the ventricular frequency is a simple factor (e.g. $\frac{1}{2}$ or $\frac{1}{3}$) of the actual frequency and the Q,R,S, and T waves are then found to follow every other (or every third) P wave. In this case the AV block is only partial and the ventricle continues to be driven by the atrial activity, though not responding to every excitation. In complete block, however, the ventricular rate is completely unrelated to the auricular rhythm.

We have already noted in earlier chapters (1 and 7) that pacemaker activity is not only found in sino-atrial tissue. It is also found in the Purkinje fibres that conduct the impulse rapidly over the ventricular surface. It is very likely therefore that the cause of continued ventricular beating in the presence of AV block is the pacemaker activity occurring in the Purkinje fibres, or in the His bundle connecting the AV node to the Purkinje fibre network. This activity is slower (e.g. 40 per minute) than SA pacemaker rates (e.g. > 60 per minute) but, as we have seen in Chapter 8, it may be increased by adrenaline. A patient with AV block, therefore, may still show sympathetic control of rhythm and increase his heart output in response to increased demands. The major problem arises simply from the fact that the frequency of beating is generally much lower than the ordinary atrial rate under any given conditions so that the work that the heart can perform is less than in a normal person.

Although it is likely that ventricular rhythm during AV block is generated by the Purkinje fibres or His bundle in mammalian hearts, it is worth noting that ventricular beating can occur in other animals, e.g. frogs, when the ventricle is isolated from the atria, even though these animals do not possess Purkinje fibres. It is clear therefore that under some circumstances normally quiescent ventricular fibres may show pacemaker activity, and it is possible that in mammals some abnormal excitation (extrasystoles) may arise from ectopic ventricular foci. In discussing these phenomena one must bear in mind the possibility that both the Purkinje tissue and ventricular tissue proper might form the site of origin of extrasystoles.

Extrasystolic excitation

Ectopic beats, by themselves, are not particularly harmful. The heart simply shows an extra contraction over and above the normal frequency. However, it is significant that ventricular fibrillation is usually preceded by ectopic beating. The occurrence of extrasystoles may be a precipitating factor in a heart that is predisposed to show fibrillation. It is therefore worth considering the nature of ectopic beats a little more closely. In particular, I shall discuss the features of an ectopic beat occuring during normal repolarization since it is during the T wave of the electrocardiogram (which corresponds to ventricular repolarization – see p. 11) that the heart is most vulnerable to fibrillation in response to ectopic beats.

We have already seen in an earlier chapter (p. 86) that the characteristics of the action potential depend on the frequency of beating. At high frequencies, the action-potential duration is decreased. One might suppose that an ectopic beat could be regarded as a sudden and transient increase in frequency so that the characteristics of the extrasystolic action potential should be those of an action potential occurring in a normal cycle of activity when the heart is beating regularly at an increased frequency. In fact, this is not so. The electrical activity of the heart (and, indeed, its mechanical activity) takes some time to adjust to a change in frequency.

We may illustrate this point most dramatically by observing the way in which fibres that are initially quiescent respond to the sudden imposition of a train of action potentials. Records of this kind obtained from Purkinje fibres are shown in Fig. 10.1. The responses to three different frequencies are illustrated and, in each case, the *transient* changes obtained when the stimulus train is started are superimposed on records obtained during *steady-state* conditions when the pulse train has continued long enough for successive action potential to be virtually identical. This way of displaying the records is particularly helpful in this case since, if the fibres adjusted almost immediately to the new frequency, the second and subsequent action potentials would all superimpose on those obtained later in the pulse train.

It is quite clear from Fig. 10.1 that this is not the case. At the beginning of each train of impulses there is an alternation of action-potential duration. This arises from the fact that the first action potential in the train is long since it follows a period of quiescence. The second action potential therefore occurs very soon after the repolarization of the first. Indeed, at high frequencies, it occurs well before repolarization is complete. The second action potential therefore occurs at a time which is very early in relation to the recovery mechanisms. The Na^+ and Ca^{2+} conductances will be subject to a high degree of inactivation while the K^+ conductance involved in repolarization will still be higher

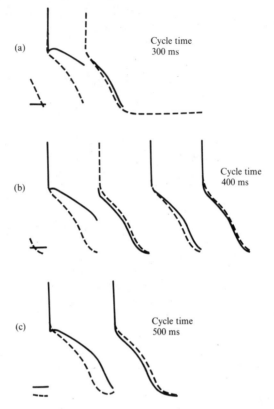

FIG. 10.1. Responses of Purkinje fibre to repetitive stimuli at three different frequencies applied after a long period of quiescence (continuous lines). The interrupted records show action potentials after sufficient stimuli are applied to reach a steady state. Note alternation in duration of initial responses. (Hauswirth, Noble, and Tsien 1972a.)

than at rest. The result is a very short action potential with a low rate of rise. The rates of rise are not shown in Fig. 10.1 but it is clear from the greatly reduced peaks of the second action potentials that the Na$^+$ conductance is low.

This phenomenon is shown more clearly in Fig. 10.2, which shows rates of rise of action potentials in Purkinje fibres elicited at various times following repolarization. The rate of rise is low when an action potential is elicited during repolarization and only fully recovers when the maximum diastolic potential is reached. This phenomenon is largely attributable to the voltage-dependence of the Na$^+$ inactivation variable

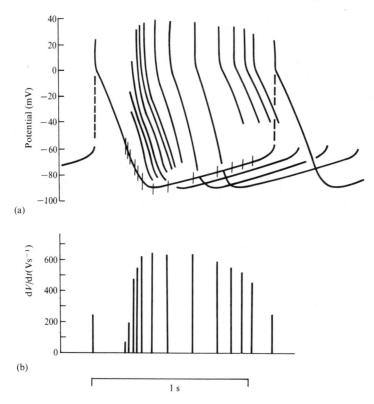

FIG. 10.2. Recovery of properties of action potentials initiated at various intervals following repolarization. (a) Action potentials recorded in spontaneously beating sheep Purkinje fibre. The responses to stimuli at various times are superimposed. (b) Rate of rise of action potential. (Weidmann 1955.)

h. As we have already seen in Chapter 4 (p. 54), the inactivation in atrial and ventricular fibres takes even longer to recover so that action potentials occurring for some time after full repolarization will conduct at abnormally low conduction velocities.

The third action potential in Fig. 10.1 follows after a much longer interval following the early repolarization of the second, so that it occurs when the recovery processes are well advanced. It is therefore long. This kind of alternation may persist for about 8–10 beats before a steady state is achieved. It is usually accompanied by a mechanical alternans in which the mechanical strength alternates.

In general, therefore, the action-potential characteristics in Purkinje fibre are mostly determined by the time elapsed since repolarization of the previous action potential (Gettes, Morehouse, and Surawicz 1972; Hauswirth, Noble, and Tsien 1972a). It should be noted also that there are substantial differences between the different parts of the heart in the way in which they respond to frequency changes. Thus Gettes, Morehouse, and Surawicz (1972) have shown that the effects of frequency on ventricular action potentials differ in significant ways from those in Purkinje fibres. Nevertheless, in all cases, the second action potential in a train at a frequency high enough for it to occur during the repolarization phase of the first action potential shows an abnormally low rate of rise. This action potential may be regarded as an extrasystole occurring during the repolarization phase in a fibre otherwise beating at a much lower frequency.

The low rate of rise and magnitude will ensure that it will conduct much more slowly (see Chapter 2, p. 38) while its shorter duration will ensure that the absolute refractory period is less than normal. These are the conditions required to generate re-excitation, which may lead to tachycardia (very high beat frequency) or to fibrillation (rapid asynchronous contraction). We may illustrate this by discussing one of the theories of tachycardia and fibrillation.

Re-entrant excitation

Sir Thomas Lewis (1925 — see also Mines (1913)) suggested that fibrillation might be attributed to a circus movement of the excitation wave. Starting at, say, point A the wave will conduct to other regions of the heart, and if one or other of the pathways of conduction returns to point A this point may receive a second excitation from the conducted wave. If it is not sufficiently refractory at this time, it may fire again so that a continuous cycle of rapid re-excitation may ensure.

In its original form this model was open to a number of objections, principally that it appeared to postulate the existence of a discrete (particular) circuit of cells or fibres that the excitation wave followed. Attempts to find such circuits generally failed. However, in 1964 Moe, Rheinboldt, and Abildskov used a computer model to show that re-entrant excitation can occur in such a way that the re-entry circuits occur more or less at random and no single circuit persists as a stable circuit. It does seem therefore that the circus theory is still plausible.

The main requirements of this theory are:

1. A circuit path length l long enough for a wave to arrive back at

its starting point with a sufficient delay to avoid arriving during the refractory period.

2. A low conduction velocity θ. Clearly, the lower θ is the shorter the path length for successful re-entrant excitation.

3. A short refractory period t_R. The minimum path length for successful re-entry also dimishes as t_R decreases. In practice, successful re-entrant excitation might occur if the time taken to conduct round the circuit, i.e. l/θ, is greater than t_R (or that $l > \theta\, t_R$).

During normal activity we must suppose that l/θ is always smaller than t_R for any possible value of l (which is, of course, limited, by the size of the heart). We begin to see here also a further function for the rapid conduction velocity generated by the Purkinje fibres. In large hearts, near-synchrony of excitation is not only desirable to ensure synchrony of contraction but also to guard against re-entrant excitation. In this connection, it is also interesting to note that the Purkinje fibre action-potential duration, and hence the refractory period, normally outlasts that of nearby ventricular cells. Since it is in the slowly conducting ventricular cells that re-entry circuits are most likely to occur under normal conditions, this may be an adaptation to ensure that any local re-entrant excitations in the ventricle do not travel back via the Purkinje fibres (Moore, Preston, and Moe 1965).

We may now return to the significance of extrasystolic excitations occurring during repolarization. As we have already noted above, these give rise to action potentials that conduct very slowly and have a short t_R. θt_R is therefore abnormally small and re-entrant excitation may occur over short path lengths. Thus, a heart in which all possible path lengths are too short to allow re-entrant excitation in response to normally occurring action potentials may show re-entrant excitation in response to an extrasystole. If there is one re-entrant circuit the result will be rapid, but nearly synchronized, beating. If the re-entrant circuits occur randomly and are numerous, the result may be asynchronous fibrillation.

Possible role of abnormal activity in Purkinje fibres

Which of these two phenomena actually occurs might depend on the state of the Purkinje fibre system since this system normally ensures rapid conduction between the various parts of the ventricle. During extrasystoles the conduction velocity decrease in the Purkinje fibres is proportionately less than in the atrial and ventricular fibres since the slow phase of recovery from Na^+ inactivation is not evident in these fibres at diastolic potentials (though it does occur at less negative potentials — see Gettes and Reuter (1974)). If the Purkinje fibre system is normal, therefore, we might expect the response to an extrasystole to be limited to a period of tachycardia or, perhaps, to the extrasystole itself.

Clearly, however, the situation will be less favourable for maintaining synchrony of contraction whenever conduction in the Purkinje fibres is severely impaired. There are various conditions in which such impairment occurs as result of depolarization of the Purkinje fibre membranes and it may be highly significant that these conditions are also known to favour the onset of fibrillation (see Surawicz 1971). Examples of these conditions are: low extracellular K^+ concentration (Carmeliet 1961; Müller 1963a); anoxia (Trautwein 1964); following treatment with ouabain (Müller 1963b); and low temperatures. All these factors may be of clinical importance in dealing with ectopic arrhythmias. Electrolyte imbalance, especially hypokalaemia, anoxia and acidosis, digitoxicity, and various conditions (congestive heart failure, myocardial ischemia) that may produce anoxia or acidosis are all regularly screened (if time is available) before deciding on treatment. It is clearly a speculation that a low membrane potential and impaired conduction (perhaps combined with low-amplitude oscillations — see Fig. 10.3) in the conducting system

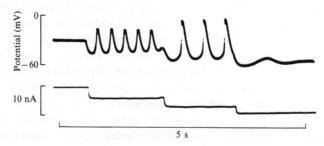

FIG. 10.3. Pacemaker activity in depolarized Purkinje fibres.

is responsible for many kinds of arrhythmia and fibrillation, but in the light of this discussion it is a speculation that deserves to be taken seriously.

The depolarizing action of low $[K^+]_0$ was discussed in the previous chapter, where we showed that it was attributable to the phenomenon of inward-going rectification. Although such rectification is present in all cardiac membranes, it is only in the Purkinje fibres that the conditions are such that large depolarizations occur in low $[K^+]_0$ (see p. 127). Thus the conducting system is particularly sensitive to loss of rapid conduction in this case. The precise mechanisms of the depolarization occurring at low temperature, in the presence of ouabain and in anoxic conditions, are not yet known but it is worth noting that, in these cases also, the Purkinje fibres appear to be most susceptible. In general, therefore, fairly small changes in ionic current flow are adequate to depolarize these fibres from the normal resting potential range (-90 mV to -80 mV) to the region of -50 mV. At this potential the Na^+ conductance is inactivated and only slowly conducted action potentials (dependent either on the Ca^{2+} current or on a small steady-state Na^+ current) may occur.

The action potentials in these conditions do not resemble those in fully polarized Purkinje fibres. The characteristic spike and plateau are lost and the wave strongly resembles action potentials obtained in sino-atrial pacemaker tissue. Moreover, as shown in Fig. 10.3, the fibres frequently show spontaneous activity that is also similar to that seen in SA pacemaker cells (compare Fig. 10.3 with Fig. 1.3(a), p. 7). It is not surprising therefore that the pacemaker potentials in this case are found to depend on the decay on the K^+ current $i_{x,1}$ rather than $i_{K^+,2}$ (Hauswirth, Noble, and Tsien 1969).

It is possible therefore that the difference between a tachycardiac response and fibrillation may depend on whether the Purkinje fibres are normally polarized and conducting rapidly, or depolarized and conducting low-amplitude waves at a much smaller velocity. It is, unfortunately, difficult to see how this question may be answered in the intact fibrillating heart since we have no techniques that allow us to record intracellular Purkinje fibre activity in these conditions. For further discussions of recent work on abnormal electrical activity the reader is referred to Biggar (1973), and Dreifus and Likoff (1973).

11 Conclusions

The measurements of ionic currents underlying excitation in cardiac muscle under controlled voltage conditions began exactly ten years ago. Despite a decade of intensive work in this field, we are still not as certain about the mechanisms of electrical activity in the heart as we may be about those in nerve. Hodgkin and Huxley required a mere three years from the first use of the voltage-clamp technique in 1949 to publishing a quantitative theory of excitation in 1952. The reasons for the slow progress in the analysis of cardiac muscle are not hard to find and have already been referred to in this book. First, as shown in Chapter 3, the voltage-clamp technique is not so easy to apply to cardiac muscle and is subject to many more sources of errors and artefacts in this case. Second, as a result of some of these difficulties it has proved difficult to arrive at reliable estimates of the magnitude of the excitatory Na^+ current (Chapter 4). Finally, the total number of ionic current mechanisms in cardiac membrane is greater than in nerve. The importance of the discovery of the Ca^{2+} current has been discussed in Chapters 5 and 6; and the roles of the different K^+ currents were discussed in Chapters 6, 7, and 8.

At the beginning of the book (Chapter 2) I indicated that I would use the 1962 model of Purkinje fibre activity, based on a simple modification of the Hodgkin–Huxley theory, as a point of reference. In subsequent chapters we have been able to see how some of the roles of the components of this model have now been attributed to one or other of the new components discovered using the voltage-clamp technique, and I have attempted to give some account of the functional reasons why the mechanisms may exist in the way they do. It may now be useful therefore to draw these accounts together in the form of a diagram showing how the 1962 model must be modified.

Quantitative models using the voltage-clamp results have in fact been formulated (McAllister, Noble, and Tsien 1975; Beeler and Reuter 1975), and the interested reader is referred to these papers for a full account of the way in which the electrical activity of Purkinje fibres and ventricular muscle may be reproduced in a mathematical form. For the purposes of this introductory account, however, I prefer to use a simpler

diagram based on re-drawing Fig. 2.6 (p. 29) so as to indicate the way
in which the conductance changes occurring during the action-potential
and pacemaker activity must be modified. This has been done in Fig.
11.1. It should be emphasized that the modifications have been drawn

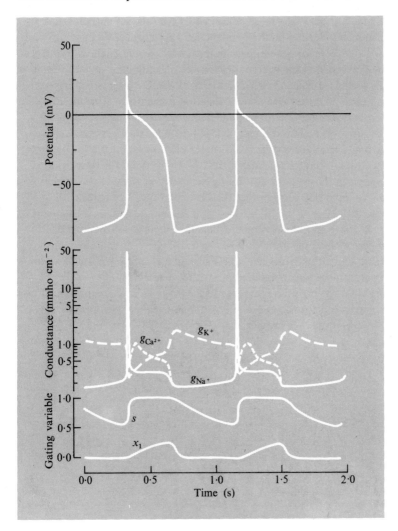

FIG. 11.1. Diagram illustrating modifications required in 1962 model (see Fig.
2.6). The inward current during the plateau has been divided into two components,
g_{Na^+} and $g_{Ca^{2+}}$. The time-dependent changes in g_{K^+} have also been divided into
two components, controlled by the gating variables, s and x_1. (Noble 1974.)

freehand; they are not the result of computer calculations.

The top diagram is the same as that given in Fig. 2.6. In the middle diagram, the 'inward' conductance has been split into two components to show how the Ca^{2+} current is activated during, and helps to maintain, the plateau. The K^+-conductance time-course is the same as that shown in Fig. 2.6 since the *overall* behaviour of the total K^+ current is not dissimilar from that in the 1962 model. It is however necessary to show two kinetic processes responsible for the K^+ current changes, and these are illustrated in the bottom diagram which shows the time-course of the gating variables s and x_1 that control the K^+ currents involved in pacemaker activity and in repolarization respectively. The *onset* of s is hardly noticed in the total conductance curve because the current $i_{K^+,2}$ it controls is activated rapidly and is very small during strong depolarizations. The time-course of s is therefore most evident in the decay of g_{K^+} responsible for pacemaker activity. Conversely, the onset of x_1 *is* evident in the onset of g_{K^+} during the plateau, but has little to contribute to the decay of g_{K^+} other than at early times during pacemaker activity.

We have seen in previous chapters that there are substantial differences between the ionic-current mechanisms in different parts of the heart and, although some of these differences are now fairly clear, it would still be too speculative to attempt diagrams similar to that of Fig. 11.1 for pacemaker activity in the SA node and other mechanisms. So far as the normal mechanism of the initiation of the heartbeat is concerned, there is still a lot of work remaining to be done.

References

ADRIAN, R.H. (1965). In discussion of Noble, D. (1965). *J. cell. comp. Physiol.* **66** (Suppl. 2), 133–4.

– (1969). Rectification in muscle membrane. *Prog. Biophys.* **19**, 339–69.

– PEACHEY, L.D. (1973). Reconstruction of the action potential of frog sartorius muscle. *J. Physiol.* **235**, 103–31.

ARMSTRONG, C.M. (1971). Interaction of tetraethylammonium ion derivatives with the potassium channel of giant axons. *J. gen. Physiol.* **58**, 413–37.

ARVANITAKI, A. (1938). *Propriétés rhythmiques de la matière vivante. II. Etude expérimentale sur le myocarde d'Helix.* Hermann, Paris.

BAKER, P.F. (1972). Transport and metabolism of calcium ions in nerve. *Prog. Biophys.* **24**, 177–223.

BARR, L., DEWEY, M.M., and BERGER, W. (1965). Propagation of action potentials and the structure of the nexus in cardiac muscle. *J. gen. Physiol.* **48**, 797–823.

BASSINGTHWAITE, J.B. and REUTER, H. (1972). Calcium movements and excitations–contraction coupling in cardiac cells. In *Electrical phenomena in the heart* (ed. de Mello), pp. 353–95. Academic Press, New York.

BAYLISS, W.M. (1913). *Principles of general physiology,* p. 667. Longmans, London.

BEELER, G.W. and REUTER, H. (1970a). Voltage clamp experiments on ventricular myocardial fibres. *J. Physiol.* **207**, 165–90.

– – (1970b). Membrane calcium current in ventricular myocardial fibres. *J. Physiol.* **207**, 191–209.

– – (1970c). The relation between membrane potential, membrane currents and activation of contraction in ventricular myocardial fibres. *J. Physiol.* **207**, 211–29.

BIGGER, J.T. (1973). Electrical properties of cardiac muscle and possible causes of cardiac anhythmias. In: *Cardiac Arrhythmias*, pp. 13–34 (Ed. L.S. Dreifus and W. Sikoff). Grune and Stratton, New York.

BOOSTEELS, S., VLEUGELS, A., and CARMELIET, E. (1970). Choline permeability in cardiac muscle cells of the cat. *J. gen. Physiol.* **55**, 602–19.

BOTTAZZI, F. (1964). Leonardo as physiologist. In *Leonardo da Vinci,* pp. 373–87. Leisure Arts, London.

BOZLER, E. (1943). The initiation of impulses in cardiac muscle. *Am. J. Physiol.* **138**, 273–82.

BRADY, A.J. (1964). Excitation and excitation–contraction coupling in cardiac muscle. *A. Rev. Physiol.* **26**, 341–56.

References

− WOODBURY, J.W. (1960). The sodium−potassium hypothesis as the basis of electrical activity in frog ventricle. *J. Physiol.* **154**, 385−407.

BROOKS, C. McC., HOFFMAN, B.F., SUCKLING, E.E., and ORIAS, O. (1955). *Excitability of the heart.* Grune and Stratton, New York.

BROOKS, C.McC. and LU, M-M. (1972). *The sino-atrial pacemaker of the Heart.* Charles C. Thomas, Illinois.

BROWN, H.F., CLARK, A., and NOBLE, S.J. (1972). Pacemaker current in frog atrium. *Nature new Biol.* **235**, 30−1.

− McNAUGHTON, P.A., NOBLE, D., and NOBLE, S.J. (1975). Adrenergic control of cardiac pacemaker currents. *Phil. Trans. R. Soc.* (In press.)

− NOBLE, S.J. (1969*a*). Membrane currents underlying delayed rectification and pacemaker activity in frog atrial muscle. *J. Physiol.* **204**, 717−36.

− − (1969*b*). A quantitative analysis of the slow component of delayed rectification in frog atrium. *J. Physiol.* **204**, 737−47.

− − (1974). Effects of adrenaline on membrane currents underlying pacemaker activity in frog atrial muscle. *J. Physiol.* **238**, 51−3.

BURDON-SANDERSON, J. and PAGE, F.J.M. (1883). On the electrical phenomena of the excitatory process in the heart of the frog and of the tortoise, as investigated photographically. *J. Physiol.* **4**, 327−38.

BURGEN, A.S.V. and TERROUX, K.G. (1953). On the negative inotropic effect in the cat's auricle. *J. Physiol.* **120**, 449−64.

CARMELIET, E. (1961). Chloride ions and the membrane potential of Purkinje fibres. *J. Physiol.* **156**, 375−88.

− and VEREECKE, J. (1969). Adrenaline and the plateau phase of the cardiac action potential. *Pflügers Arch. ges. Physiol.* **313**, 303−15.

− WILLEMS, J. (1971). The frequency dependent character of the membrane capacity in cardiac Purkinje fibres. *J. Physiol.* **213**, 85−94.

DEL CASTILLO, J. and KATZ, B. (1955). Production of membrane potential changes in the frog's heart by inhibitory nerve impulses. *Nature, Lond.* **175**, 1035.

COLE, K.S. (1949). Dynamic electrical characteristics of the squid axon membrane. *Archs. Sci. Physiol.* **3**, 253−8.

− CURTIS, H.J. (1939). Electric impedance of the squid giant axon during activity. *J. gen. Physiol.* **22**, 649−70.

CORABOEUF, E. and OTSUKA, M. (1956). L'action des solutions hyposodiques sur les potentiels cellulaires de tissu cardiaque de Mammifères. *C.r. hebd. Séanc. Acad. Sci, Paris.* **243**, 441−4.

DECK, K.A. KERN, R., and TRAUTWEIN, W. (1964). Voltage clamp technique in mammalian cardiac fibres. *Pflügers Arch. ges. Physiol.* **280**, 50−62.

− TRAUTWEIN, W. (1964). Ionic currents in cardiac excitation. *Pflügers Arch. ges. Physiol.* **280**, 65−80.

DELEZE, J. (1970). The recovery of resting potential and input resistance in sheep heart injured by knife or laser. *J. Physiol.* **208**, 547−62.

DRAPER, M.H. and WEIDMANN, S. (1951). Cardiac resting and action potentials recorded with an intracellular electrode. *J. Physiol.* **115**, 74–94.

DREIFUS, L.S. and LIKOFF, W. (1973). (Eds.) *Cardiac Arrhythmias.* Grune and Stratton, New York.

DUDEL, J., PEPER, K., RUDEL, R. and TRAUTWEIN, W. (1966). Excitatory membrane current in heart muscle (Purkinje fibres). *Pflügers Arch. ges. Physiol.* **192**, 255–73.

– RUDEL, R. (1970). Voltage and time dependence of excitatory sodium current in cooled sheep Purkinje fibres. *Pflügers Arch. ges. Physiol.* **315**, 136–58.

– TRAUTWEIN, W. (1956). *Experienta* **12**, 396.

EBASHI, S. and ENDO, M. (1968). Calcium ion and muscle contraction. *Prog. Biophy.* **18**, 123–83.

EINTHOVEN, W. (1913). Über die Deutung des Elektrokardiograms. *Pflügers Arch. ges. Physiol.* **149**, 65–86.

FITZHUGH, R. (1960). Thresholds and plateaus in the Hodgkin–Huxley nerve equations. *J. gen. Physiol.* **43**, 867–96.

FOLKOW, B. and NEIL, E. (1971). *Circulation.* Oxford University Press, New York.

FOZZARD, H.A. (1966). Membrane capacity of the cardiac Purkinje fibre. *J. Physiol.* **182**, 255–67.

FRANKENHAEUSER, B. (1962). Instantaneous potassium currents in myelinated nerve fibres of *Xenopus Laevis* investigated with voltage clamp technique. *J. Physiol.* **160**, 40–5.

FREYGANG, W.H. and TRAUTWEIN, W. (1970). The structural implications of the linear electrical properties of cardiac Purkinje fibres. *J. gen. Physiol.* **55**, 524–47.

GASKELL, W.H. (1886). The electrical changes in the quiescent cardiac muscle which accompany stimulation of the vagus nerve. *J. Physiol.* **7**, 451–2.

– (1887). On the action of muscarin upon the heart, and on the electrical changes in the non-beating cardiac muscle brought about by stimulation of the inhibitory and augmentor nerves. *J. Physiol.* **8**, 404–15.

GEORGE, E.P. and JOHNSON, E.A. (1961). Solutions of the Hodgkin –Huxley equations for squid axon treated with tetraethylammonium and in potassium rich media. *Aust. J. exp. Biol. med. Sci.* **39**, 275–94.

GESELOWITZ, D.B. and SCHMITT, D.H. (1969). Electrocardiography. In *Biological engineering* (Ed. H.P. Schwan), pp. 333–90. McGraw-Hill, New York.

GETTES, L., MOREHOUSE, N., and SURAWICZ, B. (1972). Effect of premature depolarization on action potential duration in Purkinje and ventricular fibres of the pig moderator band. Role of preceding action potential duration and proximity. *Circ. Res.* **30**, 55–66.

– REUTER, H. (1974). *J. Physiol.* **240**, 703–24.

GIEBISCH, G. and WEIDMANN, S. (1971). Membrane currents in mammalian ventricular heart muscle fibres using a voltage clamp technique. *J. gen. Physiol.* **57**, 290–6.

GILBERT, D.L. and EHRENSTEIN, G. (1969). Effect of divalent

cations on potassium conductance of squid axons: determination of surface charge. *Biophys. J.* **9**, 447–64.

GLITSCH, H.L. REUTER, H., and SCHOLZ, H. (1970). The effect of internal sodium concentration on calcium fluxes in isolated guinea-pig auricles. *J. Physiol.* **209**, 25–43.

GOLDMAN, D.E. (1943). Potential, impedance and rectification in membranes. *J. gen. Physiol.* **27**, 37–60.

GOODFIELD, G.J. (1960). *The growth of scientific physiology.* Hutchinson, London.

GOTCH, F. (1887). Inhibition of tortoise heart. *J. Physiol.* **8**, 26P.

– (1910). The succession of events in the contracting ventricle as shown by electrometer records (tortoise and rabbit). *Heart* **1**, 235–61.

HAAS, H.G., GLITSCH, H.F., and KERN, R. (1966). Kalium-fluxe und Membranpotential am Froschvorhof in Abhangigheit von der Kalium-Aussenkonzentration. *Pflügers Arch. ges. Physiol.* **288**, 43–64.

– KERN, R. (1966). Potassium fluxes in voltage clamped Purkinje fibres. *Pflügers Arch. ges. Physiol.* **291**, 69–84.

– – EINWÄCHTER, H.M., and TARR, M. (1971) Kinetics of Na inactivation in frog atria. *Pflügers Arch. ges. Physiol.* **323**, 141–57.

HALL, A.E., HUTTER, O.F., and NOBLE, D. (1963). Current–voltage relations of Purkinje fibres in sodium-deficient solutions. *J. Physiol.* **166**, 225–40.

HARRIS, C.R.S. (1973). *The heart and the vascular system in ancient Greek medicine.* Clarendon Press. Oxford.

HARVEY, W. (1628). *de Motu Cordis.* English translation by K.J. Franklin (1957). *Movement of the heart and blood in animals.* Blackwells, Oxford.

HAUSWIRTH, O., McALLISTER, R.E., NOBLE, D., and TSIEN, R.W. (1969). Reconstruction of the actions of adrenaline and calcium ions on cardiac pacemaker potentials. *J. Physiol.* **204**, 126–8P.

– NOBLE, D., and TSIEN, R.W. (1968). Adrenaline: mechanism of action on the pacemaker potential in cardiac Purkinje fibres. *Science* **162**, 916–17.

– – – (1969). The mechanism of oscillatory activity at low membrane potentials in cardiac Purkinje fibres. *J. Physiol.* **200**, 255–65.

– – – (1972a). The dependence of plateau currents in cardiac Purkinje fibres on the interval between action potentials. *J. Physiol.* **222**, 27–49.

– – – (1972b). Separation of the pacemaker and plateau components of delayed rectification in cardiac Purkinje fibres. *J. Physiol.* **225**, 211–35.

HEMPTINNE, A. de (1971a). Properties of the outward current in frog atrial muscle. *Pflügers Arch. ges. Physiol.* **329**, 321–31.

– (1971b). The frequency dependence of outward current in frog auricular fibres. *Pflügers Arch. ges. Physiol.* **329**, 332–40.

– (1973). The double sucrose gap as a method to study the electrical properties of heart cells. *Europ. J. Cardiol.* **1**, 157–62.

HILLE, B. (1968). Charges and potentials at the nerve surface. Divalent ions and pH. *J. gen. Physiol.* **51**, 221–36.

HODGKIN, A.L. (1951). The ionic basis of electrical activity in nerve and muscle. *Biol. Rev.* **26**, 339–409.

– (1958). Ionic movements and electrical activity in giant nerve fibres. *Proc. R. Soc.* B**148**, 1–37.

– KATZ, B. (1949). The effect of sodium ions on the electrical activity of the giant axon on the squid. *J. Physiol.* **108**, 37–77.

– HUXLEY, A.F. (1952). A quantitative description of membrane current and its application to conduction and excitation in nerve. *J. Physiol.* **117**, 500–44.

HOFFMAN, B.F. and CRANEFIELD, P. (1960). *Electrophysiology of the heart.* McGraw-Hill, New York.

HUTTER, O.F. (1957). Mode of action of autonomic transmitters on the heart. *Br. Med. Bull.* **13**, 176–80.

– (1961). Ion movements during vagus inhibition of the heart. In *Nervous inhibition* (ed. Florey), pp. 114–23. Pergamon Press, Oxford.

– and NOBLE, D. (1960). Rectifying properties of cardiac muscle. *Nature* **188**, 495.

– TRAUTWEIN, W. (1955), Effect of vagal stimulation on the sinus venosus of the frog's heart. *Nature, Lond.* **176**, 512.

– – (1956). Vagal and sympathetic effects on the pacemaker fibres in the sinus venosus of the heart. *J. gen. Physiol.* **39**, 715–33.

HUXLEY, A.F. (1959). Ion movements during nerve activity. *Ann. N.Y. Acad. Sci.* **81**, 221–46.

IRISAWA, H. (1972). Electrical activity of rabbit sino atrial node. In *Symposium on the electrical field of the heart* (ed. P. Rijlant). Presses Académiques Européenes, Brussels..

ISENBERG, G. and TRAUTWEIN, W. (1974). The effect of dihydro-Ouabain and lithium ions on the outward current in cardiac Purkinje fibres. Evidence for electrogenicity of active transport. *Pflügers Arch. ges. Physiol.* **350**, 41–54.

JACK, J.J.B., NOBLE, D., and TSIEN, R.W. (1975). *Electric current flow in excitable cells.* Clarendon Press, Oxford.

JOHNSON, E.A. and LIEBERMAN, M. (1971b). Heart: excitation and contraction. *A. Rev. Physiol.* **33**, 479–532.

– TILLE, J. (1961). Evidence for independence of voltage of the membrane conductance of rabbit ventricular fibres. *Nature, Lond.* **192**, 663–4.

KASSEBAUM, D.G. (1964). Membrane effects of epinephrine in the heart. *Proc. 2nd Int. Pharm. Meeting.* **5**, 95.

KEELE, C.A. and NEIL, E. (1965). *Samson Wright's applied physiology* (11th edn). Oxford University Press, London.

LENFANT, J., MIRONNEAU, J., and AKA, J.K. (1972). Activité de la fibre sino-auriculaire de grenouille: Analyse des courants membranaires responsable de l'automatisme cardiaque. *J. Physiol, Paris.* **64**, 5–18.

LEVINE, Y.K. (1972). Physical studies of membrane structure. *Prog. Biophys.* **24**, 1–74.

References

LEWIS, SIR THOMAS (1925). *Mechanism and graphic registration of the heartbeat* (3rd edn). Shaw and Sons, London.

LÜTTGAU, H.C. and NIEDERGERKE, R. (1958). The antagonism between Ca and Na ions on the frog's heart. *J. Physiol.* 143, 486–505.

MARMONT, G. (1949). Studies on the axon membrane. I. A new method. *J. cell. comp. Physiol.* 34, 351–82.

MASCHER, D. and PEPER, K. (1969). Two components of inward current in myocardial muscle fibres. *Pflügers Arch. ges. Physiol.* 307, 190–203.

McALLISTER, R.E. and NOBLE, D. (1966). The time and voltage dependence of the slow outward current in cardiac Purkinje fibres. *J. Physiol.* 186, 632–62.

– – TSIEN, R.W. (1975). Reconstruction of the electrical activity of cardiac Purkinje fibres. *J. Physiol.* (In press.)

McNUTT, N.S. and WEINSTEIN, R.S. (1973). Membrane ultrastructure at mammalian intercellular junctions. *Prog. Biophys.* 26, 45–101.

MENDEZ, C. and MOE, G.K. (1972). Atrio-ventricular transmission. In *Electrical phenomena in the heart* (ed. W.C. de Mello), pp. 263–96. Academic Press, New York.

MEREDITH, J., MENDEZ, C., MUELLER' W.J., and MOE, G.K. (1968). Electrical excitability of atrio ventricular nodal cells. *Circ. Res.* 23, 69–85.

MINES, G.R. (1913). On functional analysis by the action of electrolytes. *J. Physiol.* 46, 188–235.

MOBLEY, B.A. and PAGE, E. (1972). The surface area of sheep cardiac Purkinje fibres. *J. Physiol.* 220, 547–63.

MOE, G.K., RHEINBOLDT, W.C., and ABILDSKOV, S.A. (1964). A computer model of atrial fibrillation. *Am. Heart J.* 67, 200–20.

MONNIER, A.M. and DUBUISSON, M. (1934). *Arch. Int. Physiol.* 38, 180–1.

MOORE, E.N., PRESTON, J.B., and MOE, G.K. (1965). Durations of transmembrane action potentials and functional refractory periods of canine false tendon and ventricular myocardium. *Circ. Res.* 17, 259–73.

MORAD, M. and GOLDMAN, Y. (1973). Excitation–contraction coupling in heart muscle: membrane control of development of tension. *Prog. Biophys.* 27, 257–313.

– TRAUTWEIN, W. (1968). The effect of the duration of the action potential on contraction in the mammalian heart tissue. *Pflügers Arch. ges. Physiol.* 299, 66–82.

MÜLLER, P. (1963a). Kalium und Digitalistoxizität. *Cardiologia* 42, 176–88.

– (1963b). Digitalisuberempfindlichkeit und Digitalis resistenz. *Schweiz med. Wschr.* 33, 1038–42.

NEW, W. and TRAUTWEIN, W. (1972a). Inward membrane currents in mammalian myocardium. *Pflügers Arch. ges. Physiol.* 334, 1–23.

– (1972b). The ionic nature of slow inward current and its relation to contraction. *Pflügers Arch. ges. Physiol.* 334, 24–38.

NIEDERGERKE, R. (1963). Movements of Ca in beating ventricles of the frog. *J. Physiol.* **167**, 551–80.

NOBLE, D. (1960). Cardiac action and pacemaker potentials based on the Hodgkin–Huxley equations. *Nature, Lond.* **188**, 495–7.

— (1962*a*). A modification of the Hodgkin–Huxley equations applicable to Purkinje fibre action and pacemaker potentials. *J. Physiol.* **160**, 317–52.

— (1962*b*). Computed action potentials and their experimental basis. *Proc. int. Union Physiol. Sci.* **1**, 177–82.

— (1962*c*). The voltage dependence of the cardiac membrane conductance. *Biophys. J.* **2**, 381–93.

— (1965). Electrical properties of cardiac muscle attributable to inward-going (anomalous) rectification. *J. cell. comp. Physiol.* **66**, (Suppl. 2). 127–36.

— (1966). Applications of the Hodgkin-Huxley equations to excitable tissues. *Physiol. Rev.* **46**, 1–50.

— (1974). Cardiac action potentials and pacemaker activity. *Recent advances in physiology* (ed. R.J. Linden), pp. 1–50. Churchill, London.

— TSIEN, R.W. (1968). The kinetics and rectifier properties of the slow potassium current in cardiac Purkinje fibres. *J. Physiol.* **195**, 185–214.

— — (1969*a*). Outward membrane currents activated in the plateau range of potentials in cardiac Purkinje fibres. *J. Physiol.* **200**, 205–31.

— — (1969*b*). Reconstruction of the repolarization process in cardiac Purkinje fibres based on voltage clamp measurements of the membrane current. *J. Physiol.* **200**, 233–54.

— — (1972). The repolarization process of heart cells. In *Electrical phenomena in the heart* (ed. W.C. De Mello), pp. 133–61. Academic Press, New York.

OJEDA, C. (1971). Doctoral thesis, University of Poitiers.

ORKAND, R.K. (1968). Facilitation of heart muscle contraction and its dependence on external calcium and sodium. *J. Physiol.* **196**, 311–25.

— NIEDERGERKE, R. (1964). Heart action potential: dependence on external calcium and sodium ions. *Science* **146**, 1176–7.

— — (1966*a*). The dual effect of calcium on the action potential of the frog's heart. *J. Physiol.* **184**, 291–311.

— — (1966*b*). The dependence of the action potential of the frog's heart on external and intracellular sodium concentration. *J. Physiol.* **184**, 312–34.

OTSUKA, M. (1958). Die Wirkung von Adrenalin auf Purkinje–Fasern von Säugetieren. *Pflügers Arch. ges. Physiol.* **266**, 512–17.

PAES DE CARVALHO, A., HOFFMAN, B.F. and PAULA DE CARVALHO, M. (1969). Two components of the cardiac action potential. I. Voltage time course and the effect of acetycholine on atrial and nodal cells of the rabbit heart. *J. gen. Physiol.* **54**, 607–35.

References

PEPER, K. and TRAUTWEIN, W. (1969). A note on the pacemaker current in Purkinje fibres. *Pflügers Arch. ges. Physiol.* **309**, 356–61.

REUTER, H. (1967). The dependence of slow inward current in Purkinje fibres on the extracellular calcium concentration. *J. Physiol.* **192**, 479–92.

– (1973). Divalent cations as charge carriers in excitable membranes. *Prog. Biophys.* **26**, 1–43.

– SEITZ, N. (1968). The dependence of calcium efflux from cardiac muscle on temperature and external ion composition. *J. Physiol.* **195**, 451–70.

RINGER, S. (1883). A further contribution regarding the influence of the different constituents of the blood on the contraction of the heart. *J. Physiol.* **4**, 29–42.

RITCHIE, J.M. (1973). Energetic aspects of nerve conduction: the relationships between heat production, electrical acitivity and metabolism. *Prog. Biophys.* **26**, 147–87.

ROUGIER, O. and VASSORT, G. (1971). Interaction des ions sodium et calcium dans le courant lente et la contraction des fibres auriculaires cardiaques de grenouille. *J. Physiol., Paris* **63**, 92–3.

– – STÄMPFLI, R. (1968). Voltage clamp experiments on frog atrial heart muscle fibres with the sucrose gap technique. *Pflügers Arch. ges. Physiol.* **301**, 91–108.

– – GARNIER, D., GARGOUIL, Y-M., and CORABOEUF, E. (1969). Existence and role of a slow inward current during the frog atrial action potential. *Pflügers Arch. ges. Physiol.* **308**, 91–110.

SOMMER, J.R. and JOHNSON, E.A. (1968). Cardiac muscle: a comparative study of Purkinje fibres and ventricular fibres. *J. cell. Biol.* **36**, 497–526.

SAMOJLOFF, A. (1914). Die Vagus - und Muskarinwirkung auf die Stromkurve des Froscherzens. *Pflügers Arch. ges. Physiol.* **155**, 471–522.

SURAWICZ, B. (1971). Ventricular fibrillation. *Am. J. Cardiol.* **28**, 268–87.

TRAUTWEIN, W. (1964). Pathophysiologie des Herz Flimmerns. *Vern. dt. Ges. KreislForsch.* **30**, 40–56.

– KUFFLER, S.W. and EDWARDS, C. (1956). Changes in membrane characteristics of heart muscle during inhibition. *J. gen. Physiol.* **40**, 135–45.

– SCHMIDT, R.F. (1960). Zur Membranwirkung des Adrenalins an der Herzmuskelfaser. *Pflügers Arch. ges. Physiol.* **271**, 715–26.

TSIEN, R.W. (1970). *The kinetics of conductance changes in heart cells.* D. Phil. thesis. Oxford University.

– (1974a). Effect of epinephrine on the pacemaker potassium current of cardiac Purkinje fibres. *J. gen. Physiol.* **64**, 293–319.

– (1974b). The mode of action of chronotropic agents in cardiac Purkinje fibres. *J. gen. Physiol.* **64**, 320–42.

– GILES. W.R., and GREENGARD, P. (1972). Cyclic AMP mediates the action of adrenaline on the action potential plateau of cardiac Purkinje fibres. *Nature, new Biol.* **240**, 181–3.

VAN DER POL, B. (1926). On relaxation oscillations. *Phil. Mag.* 2, 978–92.

– VAN DER MARK, J. (1928). The heartbeat considered as a relaxation oscillation, and an electrical model of the heart. *Phil. Mag.* **6** (Suppl.) 763–75

VASSALLE, M. (1965). Cardiac pacemaker potentials at different extra- and intracellular K concentrations. *Am. J. Physiol.* **208**, 770–5.

– (1966). Analysis of cardiac pacemaker potential using a 'voltage clamp' technique. *Am. J. Physiol.* **210**, 1335–41.

– BARNABEI, O. (1971). Norepinephrine and potassium fluxes in cardiac Purkinje fibres. *Pflügers Arch. ges. Physiol.* **322**, 287–303.

VAUGHAN-WILLIAMS, E.M. (1959). The effect of changes in extra- cellur potassium concentration on the intracellular potentials of isolated rabbit atria. *J. Physiol.* **146**, 411–27.

– (1971). Biophysical background to beta-blockade. In *New perspectives in beta-blockade*, pp. 11–38.

VASSORT, G. (1973). Existence of two components in frog cardiac mechanical activity. *Europ. J. Cardiol.* **1**, 163–8.

VITEK, M. and TRAUTWEIN, W. (1971). Slow inward current and action potentials in cardiac Purkinje fibres. *Pfügers Arch. ges. Physiol.* **323**, 204–18.

WALLER, A.D. (1887). A demonstration on man of electromotive changes accompanying the heart's beat. *J. Physiol.* **8**, 229–34.

WEIDMANN, S. (1951). Effect of current flow on the membrane potential of cardiac muscle. *J. Physiol.* **115**, 227–36.

– (1952). The electrical constants of Purkinje fibres. *J. Physiol.* **118**, 348–60.

– (1955). The effect of the cardiac membrane potential on the rapid availability of the sodium carrying system. *J. Physiol.* **127**, 213–14.

– (1956). *Elektrophysiologie der Herzmuskelfaser.* Huber, Bern

– (1966). The diffusion of radiopotassium across intercalated discs of cardiac muscle. *J. Physiol.* **187**, 323–42.

– (1967). Cardiac electrophysiology in the light of recent morpho- logical findings. *Harvey Lect.* **61**, 1–15.

WEST, T.C. (1961). Effects of chronotropic influences on subthreshold oscillations in the sino-atrial nodes. In *Specialized tissues of the heart* (eds. A. Paes de Carvalho, W.C. de Mello, and B. Hoffman), pp. 81–94. American Elsevier, New York.

– (1955). Auricular cellular potentials: ultramicroelectrode recording of drug effects on nodal and extranodal regions. *Fedn Proc. Fedn Am. Socs exp. Biol.* **14**, 160.

WHITTERIDGE, G. (1971). *William Harvey and the circulation of the blood.* MacDonald, London.

WINEGRAD, S. and SHANES, A.M. (1962). Calcium flux and contractility in guinea-pig atria. *J. gen. Physiol.* **45**, 371–94.

WOODBURY, J.W. (1961). Voltage and time-dependent membrane

References

conductance changes in cardiac cells. In *Biophysics of physiological and pharmacological actions* (ed. A.M. Shanes). A.A.A.S., New York.

Index

Index

conductance, 20; *see also* calcium
current; sodium current
conducting tissue, 4
conduction velocity,
arrhythmias, role in, 131
AV node, in, 38
Purkinje fibres, in, 38, 138
sodium conductance, relation to,
57
contraction,
adrenaline, effect of, 67
action potential, relation to, 9
calcium ions, role in, 64, 128
frequency, effect of, 86
initiation of, 64
potassium ions, effect of, 128
sodium ions, effect of, 128

depolarization,
calcium current, role of, 49
plateau, independence of, 63
potassium ions, and, 128
rate of, 30, 36, 57, 135
sodium current, role of, 49, 54
digitalis, *see* cardiac glycosides

ectopic beats, 132
electrical conduction, 34
electrocardiogram (ECG), 2
action potentials, relation to, 10
AV block, during, 131
electrochemical potential gradient, 19
electrogenic pump current, 17, 112,
121
epinephrine, *see* adrenaline
equilibrium potentials, 19, 95
extrasystoles, 132, 137

fibrillation, 131
acidosis, role of, 138
anoxia, role of, 138
circus theory of, 136
ectopic beats, role of, 133
potassium ions, role of, 138
frequency,
acetyl choline, effect of, 105
adrenaline, effect of, 107
duration of action potential,
effect on, 86, 133
rate of rise, effect on, 135
temperature, effect of, 90

gating mechanisms, 20, 22

'healing over', 40
hearth block (AV block), 4, 6, 101,
131, 132
His bundle, 5, 132
Hodgkin–Huxley theory, 22, 28, 89

inactivation, 25, 54
injury potential, 104
intracellular resistance, 32, 37
inward-going rectification, 21, 27, 30
background current, in, 119
pacemaker activity, role in, 95
plateau, role in, 74
potassium ions, effects of, 122
resting potential, role in, 127
ionic concentrations, 18
ionic current, 24; *see also* calcium
current, potassium current,
sodium current

leak current, 118
lithium ions, 17
local circuit current, 33

manganese ions, 60, 62
membrane capacitance, 36, 38, 49
deep, 50
surface, 50, 57
membrane current, 35, 37; *see also*
calcium current, potassium
current, sodium current
membrane structure, 35

nexus, 33
Nernst equation, 19
'notch', 71

ouabain, *see* cardiac glycosides
outward-going rectification, 20

pacemaker activity during AV block,
6, 132
pacemaker potential, 6
acetyl choline, effect of, 106
adrenaline, action of, 107
atrial muscle, in, 99
reconstruction of, 96
temperature, effect of, 90
pacemaker range,
atrial fibres, 8, 91
Purkinje fibres, 8, 90
plateau, 8
calcium ions, role of, 62